Integrating Wellness

Into Your

Disease Management

Programs

Second Edition

John H. Harris III, M.Ed., FAWHP
Dexter W. Shurney, MD, MBA, MPH

John H. Harris III, M.Ed., FAWHP, Author

Dexter W. Shurney, MD, MBA, MPH, Author

Les Masterson, Managing Editor

Matt Cann, Group Publisher

Patrick Campagnone, Cover Designer

Mike Mirabello, Senior Graphic Artist

Crystal Beland, Layout Artist

Audrey Doyle, Copyeditor

Liza Banks, Proofreader

Darren Kelly, Books Production Supervisor

Susan Darbyshire, Art Director

Jean St. Pierre, Director of Operations

Advice given is general. Readers should consult professional counsel for specific legal, ethical, or clinical questions.

Arrangements can be made for quantity discounts. For more information, contact:

HCPro, Inc.

P.O. Box 1168

Marblehead, MA 01945

Telephone: 800/650-6787 or 781/639-1872

Fax: 781/639-2982

E-mail: *customerservice@hcpro.com*

Visit HCPro at its World Wide Web sites:
www.hcpro.com and **www.hcmarketplace.com**

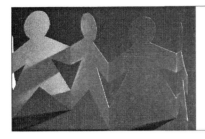

Contents

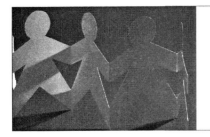

About the Authors

John H. Harris III, M.Ed., FAWHP

John H. Harris III, M.Ed., FAWHP, is chief wellness officer and senior vice president at Healthways, a company specializing in health management in the corporate and health plan sectors. Harris was the cofounder of Harris HealthTrends, Inc., an entrepreneurial corporation specializing in the prevention of disease and the reduction of healthcare costs. He received a bachelor's of science degree from Grand Valley State University in 1977, and a master's in education degree from The University of Toledo in 1982.

Harris is a fellow in the Association for WorkSite Health Promotion, and serves on numerous health-related boards internationally. Harris speaks internationally, has been the author of numerous publications on employee health, and has served as a consultant to many Fortune 500 companies.

Dexter W. Shurney, MD, MBA, MPH

Dexter W. Shurney, MD, MBA, MPH, senior vice president and chief medical officer of Healthways, has an extensive background in healthcare management and consulting. Prior to joining Healthways, Shurney served as a key strategist in health policy for the biotechnology company Amgen Inc. In addition, he is the former chief medical officer and vice president of medical affairs for Blue Cross Blue Shield of Michigan.

Shurney currently serves on Tennessee Gov. Phil Bredesen's Diabetes Prevention and Health Improvement Board and on the boards of the American College of Medical Quality and the Integrated Benefits Institute.

Shurney is board-certified in preventive medicine. He received his bachelor's degree from Loma Linda University and his medical degree from Howard University, Washington, D.C. He holds graduate degrees in business and in public health from the University of Detroit/Mercy College of Business and from the Medical College of Wisconsin, respectively.

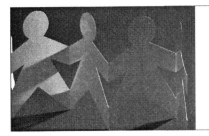

Introduction

In the past few years, healthcare costs in the United States have soared to a record $2 trillion. As these expenses continue to escalate, more companies are searching for ways to curb these costs while keeping their employees—and their bottom line—healthy. This has resulted in a paradigm shift for employers who are now focusing on prevention and disease management as one way to trim costs and support employee health.

In fact, employer interest in employee health and wellness has surged in the past few years. Companies large and small have begun to develop and launch a variety of wellness programs and health initiatives as a way to address these issues. These wellness initiatives offer everything from weight loss and smoking cessation programs to health and biometric screenings, coaching sessions, and programs designed specifically to manage chronic diseases and pain. The personal wellness options offered to employees today have never been greater.

This concept of personalizing wellness is a direct result of employers embracing the critical relationship between health, productivity, and healthcare costs. Smart businesses, which are leading the charge in supporting personalized health through disease management and wellness programs, are driving a new emerging model of healthcare, one based on the modern needs of today's workers.

In fact, the future of disease management is irrevocably tied to wellness and the larger health management movement. And creating an effective and well-accepted health management program requires careful planning and execution to ensure it remains on the cutting edge of this important trend.

You can build a successful health management initiative, and HCPro's *Integrating Wellness Into Your Disease Management Programs, Second Edition* can show you how. This updated second edition goes well beyond the content of its predecessor, offering strategies and practical solutions that focus on the ways to create and implement successful health management initiatives. Each chapter is packed with information that will help lead to a successful health and wellness program implementation and launch.

Wellness programs today can have true business impact, but only if they offer effective programs that satisfy the needs of both employers and employees. The call for incorporating disease management and wellness offerings into a larger health management effort has increased exponentially in recent years. Companies must find ways to keep up with the demand while incorporating creative methods to engage employees in adopting healthy habits. Developing a companywide health management plan can be the answer, and *Integrating Wellness Into Your Disease Management Programs, Second Edition* is chock-full of information to show you how to do it.

Specifically, the book provides new strategies on how to

- Craft wellness disease management program

- Gain senior executive support

- Tailor the right programs for all employees

- Use new technology and tools available for maximum impact

- Implement your program for greatest success

The book also highlights the most effective ways to fund and evaluate your health management program so that you gain the most support while effectively utilizing your program's investment effectively. *Integrating Wellness Into Your Disease Management Programs, Second Edition* will help your organization discover ways to improve health while saving money (in both productivity and health costs). Additionally, the book will highlight actionable steps, such as:

- Implementing health management programs using case examples of successful examples from peers

- Creating smart predictive models that combine claims data review with health surveys to find people who are both at risk and willing to make a change

- Developing effective coaching techniques and creating incentives that spark healthy living

Integrating Wellness Into Your Disease Management Programs will also provide the most up-to-date information on the legalities of launching programs, along with information on how to revitalize a program that may have grown stagnant.

The concept of personalized healthcare is gaining momentum with employers and employees alike. Some predict that in a few short years, it will be uncommon for companies not to offer a health and wellness program. In fact, a survey of more than 500 major U.S. employers by Hewitt Associates found that the number of companies using wellness and disease management programs has increased from 73% in 2004 to 83% in 2005. By offering health initiatives, employers are demonstrating that they are serious about keeping employees well, as well as changing the unhealthy behavior, which lies at the root of most chronic disease.

If you are thinking of developing a health management program in your organization, or if you'd like to breathe new life into an existing program, why not start with a solid, fundamental plan to do so?

Integrating Wellness Into Your Disease Management Programs, Second Edition will show you how to launch your program successfully, deliver cost-efficient programs, and maximize participation. Health management goes beyond finding people who are at risk or who already have a disease or diseases. A comprehensive program reaches people at all levels of health and either keeps them healthy or improves their health by connecting them to effective health coaching, targeted e-mails, interactive Web sites, and other engaging programs.

This book will show you these approaches that have proven to be most effective and engaging. Armed with the strategic information offered here, you can build a practical health management program that will attract employees, improve productivity, and lower healthcare costs. With the right information, your health management program can endure for years, while accomplishing the ongoing wellness goals you have established for your company.

Chapter 1

The Need for Disease Management and Wellness Programs

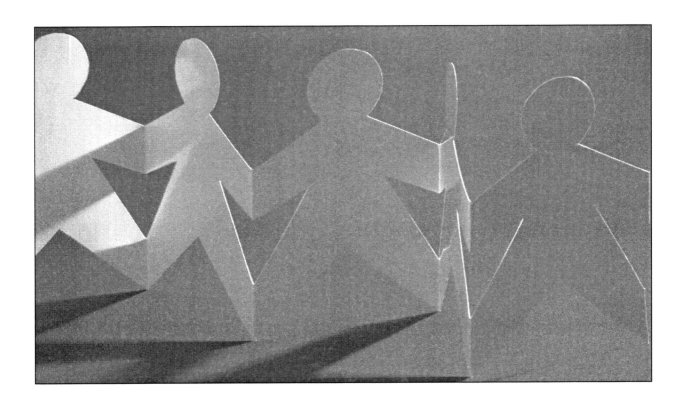

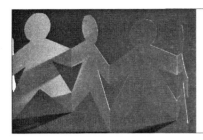

The Need for Disease Management and Wellness Programs

With medical costs spiraling out of control, more U.S. companies are being forced to shift the cost burden to their employees and dependents and make budgeting cuts that are not advantageous to their business. As a result, organizations large and small are realizing that finding cost-effective, workable solutions to the healthcare crisis will keep both employees—and the bottom line—healthy.

As a result, employer interest in the health and wellness of employees has surged in the past few years.

And with good reason.

The Statistics Tell the Story

According to the National Business Group on Health, the nation's total healthcare bill reached a staggering $2.16 trillion in 2006, an increase from $1.4 trillion in 2001. As a comparison, healthcare expenditures were $27 billion in 1960. Of the $2.16 trillion in 2006, $745 billion was paid by private insurance payments, covered primarily by businesses.

American workers are also feeling the pinch as they now spend an average of $8,748 per year in healthcare costs. In 2007, a family of four was paying $12,106 in health insurance for the year. Businesses spend an additional $6,852 per employee. According to the Kaiser Family Foundation and the Health Research & Educational Trust, premiums for employer-sponsored health insurance programs increased an average of 6% in 2007, and experts expect healthcare expenditures to reach $4 trillion by 2015. The Centers for Disease Control and Prevention (CDC) reports that for every 3 cents U.S. society spent on prevention, it spent 97 cents for curative treatment.

These alarming statistics and escalating costs point to many factors, the most significant of which is chronic disease—and its related costs. The CDC noted in its comprehensive report, *The Power of Prevention*, that the United States spends more on healthcare than any other country. Yet, the United States is ranked a mere 37th on the global list of best overall healthcare according to the 2007 World Health Organization report. More than 1.7 million Americans die of a chronic disease each year, which accounts for about 70% of deaths. Smoking-related health problems costs businesses $80 billion per year in lost productivity; poor nutrition costs another $9 billion. In 2002, the estimated nationwide cost for diabetes was a whopping $132 billion.

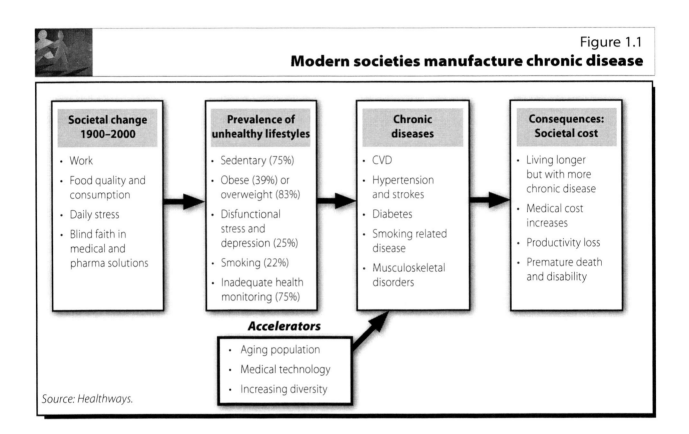

Figure 1.1

Modern societies manufacture chronic disease

Societal change 1900–2000	Prevalence of unhealthy lifestyles	Chronic diseases	Consequences: Societal cost
• Work • Food quality and consumption • Daily stress • Blind faith in medical and pharma solutions	• Sedentary (75%) • Obese (39%) or overweight (83%) • Disfunctional stress and depression (25%) • Smoking (22%) • Inadequate health monitoring (75%)	• CVD • Hypertension and strokes • Diabetes • Smoking related disease • Musculoskeletal disorders	• Living longer but with more chronic disease • Medical cost increases • Productivity loss • Premature death and disability

Accelerators

- Aging population
- Medical technology
- Increasing diversity

Source: Healthways.

Author Paul Hemp, in an article in the *Harvard Business Review*, noted that depressed employees cost U.S. employers more than $35 billion per year in reduced performance. On-the-job pain, including back pain, headaches, and arthritis, costs employers almost another $47 billion per year in productivity loss. Obesity has also become a major problem. According to the *Journal of Occupational and Environmental Medicine*, obesity-related medical claims account for 2.8% of all medical costs for adults aged 19 to 64.

Among overweight and obese adults, each one-unit increase in body mass index yields an additional $119.70 in annual medical costs and $82.60 in drug costs. To put the costs in real dollars, one study illustrated how chronic conditions have cost The Dow Chemical Company more than $100 million annually in lost productivity for its U.S. work force.

Not surprisingly, employers struggling to ease their pain are increasingly looking beyond the next treatment management option to how to address the root cause. A growing body of research shows that common, modifiable health risks, such as tobacco use, poor nutrition, stress, obesity, and lack of exercise, significantly impact employers' direct and indirect health costs. These costs also include lost productivity in the form of absenteeism and presenteeism, and workers' compensation claims.

Given all of this, business leaders are not waiting for politicians to endlessly debate the issues. Instead, they are taking a proactive stance in getting their employees healthy—and keeping them healthy. With numerous studies underscoring the significant cost associated with poor lifestyle, smart companies recognize that much of this could be avoided if workers and their dependents lived healthier lifestyles.

Further, they understand that even small percentages of improvement can yield significant cost savings. Gone are the days of simply hoping that employees will keep themselves healthy with little support from employers. Employers are finding they need a comprehensive health management program to support the creation of and maintenance of a strong work force. Improvement in human capital assets will ultimately yield a strategic business advantage.

A comprehensive health management program can produce numerous employee benefits, and show a company's dedication to and care for its employees and their families. With such a program in place, workers will respond with a more positive attitude toward the company and a stronger commitment to its mission. Employees will also achieve a greater sense of enjoyment from their work and thereby will become more productive and goal-oriented.

With so much at stake, and so much to gain or lose, organizations across the United States are casting a critical eye toward the development and implementation of more comprehensive, companywide health management programs.

The New Healthcare Model

As smart businesses lead the charge in supporting disease management and wellness, a new model of healthcare is emerging, one based on the modern needs of today's workers. Employers agree with the findings of the Boston Consulting Group that the proactive management or prevention of chronic conditions represents the single largest opportunity to improve health and contain healthcare costs.

Wellness programs are a good strategy, offering employees everything from weight loss and smoking cessation programs, to blood pressure and diabetes screenings, to programs designed to specifically manage chronic diseases and pain. The options are many, and we will explore them further in future chapters, but the common objective is to create and to maintain good health for every employee to the best extent possible.

A survey by the International Foundation of Employee Benefit Plans found that:

- 62% of organizations surveyed offer wellness initiatives

- 68% offer health risk assessments (HRAs)

- More than 80% have average participation of 50% or less

- 73% offered incentives for participation

The good news is that, overall, these programs are paying off. According to the CDC's *Partnership for Prevention*, every dollar a company invests in an effective wellness program returns a $3.50 savings in healthcare costs. Companies with these programs also reported a 28% reduction in absenteeism, a 30% reduction in workers' compensation and disability claims, and a 26% drop in healthcare costs.

Part of the success of these programs has resulted from tailoring wellness to the individual, with a personalized focus. Also, because employers are beginning to understand the critical relationship between health and productivity and cost, they are offering programs and incentives that were

unheard of just a few years ago. Many predict that in a few short years, it will be uncommon for companies not to have some kind of employee health and wellness program driven by some form of incentive or disincentive.

Health management programs have been shown to provide a variety of health benefits—for both employees and employers. These include a competitive recruiting advantage, reduction of absenteeism and turnover, higher productivity, improved morale, and strengthened goodwill toward management. Employees who actively engage in wellness and disease management programs show improvement in overall well-being, physical and mental stamina, increased job satisfaction, higher productivity, and better interpersonal relations, both on and off the job.

According to a *Workplace Wellness Report* by the Alexander Hamilton Institute, Inc. (AHI), participation in employer-sponsored wellness programs is at an all-time high. AHI cites a 2006 Principal Financial Well-Being Index survey of companies employing 10 to 1,000 employees that found that:

- 79% of employees (as compared to 68% in 2005) participated in on-site health screenings

- 65% of employees implemented a personalized action plan for high-risk conditions, up from 45% in 2005

- 60% of employees (as compared to 38% in 2005) took advantage of fitness facilities when offered this benefit

A Multifaceted Approach

Many experts in wellness and disease management agree that a program with a mixture of internal and external components works best. This approach, of developing an internal program while partnering with an outside firm capable of providing many wellness components, can have a potent impact on the success of your health management program. We will delve further into the best ways to set up and launch your program for maximum effectiveness in future chapters.

After conducting a 2007 survey to gain insight about consumer viewpoints on health, wellness, and medical insurance, Guardian, a leading provider of employee and voluntary benefits, found that larger employers are more likely to embrace wellness programs. The survey, *Benefits & Behavior: Spotlight on Group Medical*, found that:

- 82% of small employers, 90% of midsize employers, and 99% of large employers see value in implementing wellness programs. However, only 57% of the small businesses that value wellness programs have implemented some type of plan.

- 79% of the midsize businesses and 90% of large businesses that value wellness programs have one in place.

The survey also showed that:

- Three in 10 employees currently participate or have participated in a wellness program in the past three years

- 35% of employees report access to wellness programs at work; half of those who believe that they have access at work are currently enrolled in a program

- 68% of employees believe that incentives, such as cash, gifts, and extra vacation days, can help them to strengthen their willpower to adopt healthier behaviors, such as exercising, eating properly, and kicking smoking habits

- Two-thirds of all employees, and 85% of those who are currently enrolled or have participated in a wellness program in the past three years, said these programs are very effective in promoting good health

"Workplace-based wellness programs are growing in popularity with employers, largely to promote prevention and early intervention as a means to help control the cost of healthcare," said Tim Bireley, vice president, Group Medical, Guardian.

"With only a third of employees reporting that wellness programs are available at their jobs, employers and the benefits industry have to do a better job of increasing awareness about these programs. There is also an enormous opportunity to educate small and midsize business owners about the benefits of wellness initiatives. If most employees at companies large and small were actively participating in wellness programs, we might see a significant decline in the cost of medical care in the United States."

A History of Disease Management

Typically, disease management programs have focused on preventing hospitalizations and invasive procedures by keeping conditions from worsening and patients from experiencing complications of their illnesses or treatments. According to DMAA: The Care Continuum Alliance (formerly the Disease Management Association of America), and as reported in The Boston Consulting Group's report, *Realizing the Promise of Disease Management*, disease management programs routinely:

- Deploy practice guidelines focused on proven treatments

- Engage physicians and support-service providers in devising and maintaining a plan of care for the patient

- Empower patients to play a role in their own care by providing them with self-management education, which may address prevention, behavior modification, and compliance

- Include process and outcome measurements for assessing clinical, quality-of-life, and economic outcomes on an ongoing basis

It's impossible to pinpoint the precise moment when disease management came into being, but it came to the forefront with the commercial launch of blood glucose monitoring systems and hospital-based programs such as American Healthways (now called Healthways) for diabetics in the early 1980s. This started a trend of organizing care on a disease-specific basis with emerging health outcomes, which was particularly appealing to specialized providers. In fact, HMOs such as Harvard Community Health Plan and Kaiser Permanente embraced the concept quickly. Using this disease-specific model as a basis, several insurance companies, HMOs, and provider organizations began testing the parameters of disease management in the late 1980s.

The momentum for disease-specific programs picked up pace in the 1990s, when pharmaceutical companies introduced "disease-state" disease management programs to health plans and employers. They embraced the concepts and popularized the term. Payers, however, took a skeptical view of pharmaceutical-sponsored disease management programs, especially when the companies had incentives to offer their own brand drugs. The perceived move to capture and expand market share by pharmaceutical companies made many in the healthcare field suspect.

Concurrently, some companies also began offering "soft-touch" wellness initiatives, such as health-related newsletters, and, perhaps, a discounted gym membership or a nutritional guidance class. These products were seldom specific to a particular audience and were known more informally as "spray and pray" wellness. These soft-touch approaches generally tended to focus primarily on the objective of creating awareness. Many employees did not participate, and those who did were often the ones already living healthier lifestyles. This is not to say that such programs do not have a role, particularly as components within a more comprehensive approach to the problem. By the end of the 1990s, without a groundswell of support, many wellness programs and pharmaceutical-sponsored disease management programs were quietly dropped.

Companies explore wellness

Here are just a few examples of companies that have seriously implemented health management programs:

- CIGNA launched its Healthy Life initiative in 2006, offering HRAs, biometric screenings, and health coaches to its 24,000 workers. The aim of the program is to give personalized, one-on-one attention to employees, who may be facing myriad health concerns. Because of the large numbers of employees grappling with obesity and diabetes, the company also took a look at its cafeteria offerings and eliminated high-calorie, high-fat, fried foods and replaced them with healthier, lower-calorie items. This change included company vending machines, which now offer nuts, as an alternative to candy bars.

- CVS Caremark provides its 190,000 employees across the United States with an assortment of wellness programs, including the Weight Watchers, NutriSystem, and Jenny Craig weight loss programs. According to CVS Caremark, employees who enrolled in its health management program decreased their emergency room visits by 4% and hospitalizations by 12%. The number of employees who enrolled in exercise programs jumped to 80% from 62% and 92% reported having their cholesterol checked.

> ## Companies explore wellness (cont.)
>
> - For the past 15 years, GlaxoSmithKline has been at the forefront of employee wellness, recognizing that employers play a big role in getting employees to maintain their healthy lifestyles. The corporation covers the entire cost of preventive care for its 25,000 U.S. employees, including physicals and well-child visits. It will also pay the full cost for any employee who wants to stop smoking, and it will pay $100 cash to employees who take an HRA survey.
>
> - Aetna also offers its employees health risk assessments, paying up to $600 to employees who agree to take the assessments. It also offers weight and health management programs. One of its newest programs, a 16-week *Get Active Aetna* exercise program, resulted in 53% of the insurance giant's 26,000 employees walking the equivalent of 3 million miles. This equated to 852,000 hours of exercise.
>
> - Sanofi-aventis makes multiple health resources available to approximately 16,000 employees in its 14 U.S. locations. These resources include clinics at each of its major sites, prostate, blood pressure, and skin cancer screenings, healthy food selections in its cafeterias, nutrition and exercise programs, and an annual flu shot drive.

However, a subtle sea change was taking place in the 1990s that would have a revolutionary impact on the disease management and wellness field of the future: Visionaries, many of whom were also entrepreneurs, set their sights on the largely underserved markets for disease management and wellness and began offering an assortment of health solutions to companies large and small. By combining the expertise of healthcare management, and research, technology, and data mining, these entrepreneurs quickly developed an entire disease management services sector.

A new model of disease management is now being established. Unlike in the past, today many payers have widely embraced disease management initiatives that are much broader in scope and are slowly evolving away from siloed, disease-specific programs. Today's programs are more encompassing, focusing on a holistic approach to care that helps to reduce the population's overall risk.

By offering biometric medical screenings along with online health assessments, health coaches, and even on-site medical clinics, employers are demonstrating they are serious about keeping employees well, and changing unhealthy behavior, which lies at the root of most disease. Well more than 50% of chronic illness is preventable and is associated with poor choices and unhealthy behavior. Effectively changing behavior requires a focus on prevention and lifestyle management, rather than treatment alone, and health management programs today are attempting to light the way.

Because most of the $2 trillion spent on healthcare last year was exhausted on diagnosis and treatment, a focus on disease management and disease prevention is the new mathematical model, and companies are beginning to understand and embrace the equation. According to the Society for Human Resource Management, in 2006, 62% of employers offered a wellness program and another 6% planned to implement one.

To address this prevention trend, employers are beginning to offer employees a combination of wellness options designed to address the whole person, including the support of employees who are well and want to remain that way. Keeping the healthy well is the aim. By providing programs that support the healthy, change the behaviors of persons at risk, and manage the diseases of persons with chronic conditions, companies can provide wellness support across the organization. That has become the driving engine in today's health management environment.

The approach seems to be working. For instance, according to ComPsych Corp., in 2006, 30% of U.S. workers reported having a healthy diet, up from 25% in 2005. At the same time, those describing themselves as "very overweight" decreased from 24% to 22%, and those describing their workplace as "not healthy" declined from 40% to 32%.

Making a Difference

Companies can help lead the wellness charge by taking a leadership role in implementing and supporting health management programs within their organizations. This book is intended to provide the information needed to launch a successful and enduring health management program, one that employees will enthusiastically utilize. Now is the time to develop such a program, because cost-shifting and cost-containment strategies have failed to stem the growing monetary and chronic disease problems in healthcare. To maintain a competitive advantage, companies must join forces with employees and be proactive in addressing the root cause of their growing healthcare dilemma.

Organizations are not only getting the message, but embracing it. DMAA: The Care Continuum Alliance (formerly the Disease Management Association of America), as reported in The Boston Consulting Group's report, *Realizing the*

Promise of Disease Management, found that the number of companies that sell disease management services have grown rapidly over the past decade, and the Disease Management Purchasing Consortium estimates that disease management operating revenue increased from about $78 million in 1997 to almost $1.2 billion in 2005—equaling a 40% compound annual rate of growth.

Bucks Consultants, a leading human resources and benefits consulting firm, analyzed responses from 555 organizations representing almost 7 million employees. In its report, *WORKING WELL: A Global Survey of Health Promotion and Workplace Wellness Strategies*, the firm found wellness programs prevalent in the United States, with 86% of respondents offering some form of health management program. They also found that one in five employers outside the United States provided wellness programs.

Interestingly, the goals that companies set for these programs varied around the world. Whereas U.S. companies placed healthcare cost reduction as a top goal, Canadian employers cited employee attraction and retention as their primary objective. In Europe, reduction of employee absences because of sickness or disability was a top goal. Other countries reported seeking improved workplace morale and superior worker productivity.

These differences are most likely because of the fact that the US is the only country in which the employers pay most of the healthcare bill. However, from these results, it is evident that there are many values of health management programs, regardless of the payment system.

The report also found that among U.S. respondents, 33% reported a reduction in healthcare cost trend rates attributed to their wellness initiatives; some reported a reduction of 2% to 5% per year.

Web portals, online programs, and personal health records were found to be the fastest-growing components of wellness programs. Employee health fairs and workplace wellness competitions were also reported to be on the rise.

Stepping Up to the Plate on Wellness

As we mentioned, a host of companies across the United States have developed and implemented wellness programs. In fact, a survey of more than 500 major U.S. employers by Hewitt Associates found that the number of companies using wellness and disease management programs increased from 73% in 2004 to 83% in 2005. The survey further reported that 30% of employers offer incentives to encourage employee participation in wellness programs, which is up from 21% in 2004.

The Society for Human Resource Management's 2005 Benefits Survey found that 62% of respondents offer a wellness program, resources, and information, which is up from 56% in 2004.

As medical costs continue to escalate, disease management and wellness programs are now strategies whose time has come. More companies are finding creative ways to keep their employees healthy, and in doing so, are reducing health-related costs.

This book shares ideas and best approaches for developing and launching your own companywide health management initiative. Armed with a strategic implementation and evaluation plan, you can build an effective health management effort that will attract your employees, while showing real results in better health and cost impact. Aptly done, your health management initiative can be something that endures for years and meets the goals you set for your organization and its employees.

Paving the way to a healthier and more productive future for your employees is the right thing to do, and the benefits of doing so extend beyond direct healthcare costs. Improvements are often found in the areas of productivity, employee retention, safety, and even workers' compensation.

Crafting Your Organization's Health Management Program

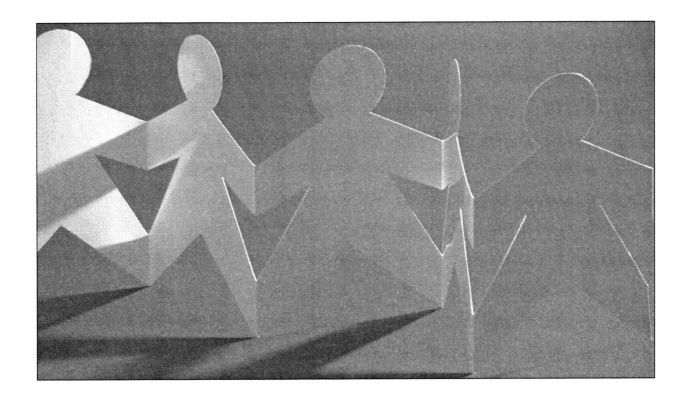

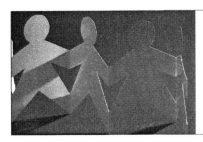

Crafting Your Organization's Health Management Program

One of the best ways in which to create an effective health management program is to take a holistic approach, allowing each component to work in relationship with the others. When you create a new health management program, you must take many factors into consideration. We will explore what some of these factors are and how to address them throughout this book. This chapter provides a brief overview of some of the components to consider when launching a companywide health management effort. By taking the following steps, you can help to streamline the planning and launching process.

Establish a Steering Committee

Setting up an initial steering committee will help keep the program planning process focused and on track. With the myriad tasks required to create and implement an effective health management program, a steering committee can effectively schedule planning meetings, analyze existing information, review problems, create timelines, formulate solutions, and, on the whole, keep the process moving.

The steering committee should be composed of representatives throughout the organization, including senior management, who will be responsible for executive decisions, budgeting, and contracting; and middle managers, department heads, and various other key employees, who are supportive of the effort and can lend valuable expertise to the process. The committee may also want to select an outside consultant with expertise in health management program planning to help facilitate the development of an overall strategic plan.

It is important to keep in mind that the larger the committee, the more difficult it may be for people to meet and make decisions. If at all possible, keep the number of committee participants to no more than eight people.

Outline the Planning Process

Effective planning will help to ensure the success of your health management program, and the right approach to this process will be crucial. Having a plan in place will also help to support any necessary changes in company policy that will be necessary to support the organization's health management effort.

During this initial planning phase, it is recommended that the steering committee perform a "culture audit." This audit will help to determine the existing extent to which the workplace or company culture supports health of employees and where improvements need to be made. We will cover this in more depth in Chapter 4.

Surveys, or companywide focus groups, should also be conducted to raise awareness of and receptivity to health management efforts. By better understanding perceptions of health and the changes needed throughout the organization, you will be able to best focus your health management efforts. Surveys and focus groups can also help to establish the program's direction for use during the development of an overall strategic plan.

Your planning process should also include interviews with various departments and other stakeholders for their input and feedback. People tend to support efforts they helped formulate. The vital feedback and opinions the committee receives will not only help bring cohesion to the planning process, but also can yield valuable insights and create preliminary buy-in to the program.

The steering committee should also review existing information available—both internally and

externally. Internal information might include previous surveys on health benefits, aggregate health risk assessment (HRA) reports, claims data and healthcare utilization studies, existing company policies (e.g., smoking in the workplace, flextime, etc.), and obvious cultural norms, such as the food offered in the cafeteria, safety-friendly ways to be active near company premises, and food served at company functions. Externally, becoming familiar with the successful programs and approaches that other companies have launched will help the committee be in a better place to organize, plan, and implement its own course of action.

Early in the process the committee should discuss where to locate the wellness program within the corporate structure and who will provide oversight. Will human resources drive the program? Or will the creation of a new department make the program more effective? It's critical to determine where the health management program will report. Some programs thrive, and others never reach their potential, depending on where they are placed within the organization.

Once you have determined an initial direction for the health management effort, you should formulate a strategic plan of action that includes a vision statement, goals, and objectives. Programs that specifically outline an overarching vision statement for the health management initiative are more successful. Companies that effectively communicate the overall vision to employees also have better participation.

The same holds true for goals and objectives. By outlining goals in a concrete manner, as well as the objectives that must be met to succeed, the intent of the program is clear, making it more likely employees and their dependents will become engaged. The ultimate plan should provide many ways for employees and dependents to participate and be supported on their own terms, using the medium of their choice, for efforts they are ready and prepared to undertake.

Once the initial strategic plan is in place, have it approved by the CEO, executive management, and any other important constituencies who may be impacted by the health management initiative. This approval process will help gain overall support of the program, while ensuring that all stakeholders have a chance to contribute to the overall design.

Determine Executive Management and Employee Support

As we mentioned before, the support of executive management, along with strong employee interest, will be critical in launching and maintaining your companywide health management program. Without the support of both, the program may never get off the ground or, worse yet, may languish from lack of participation.

The support of executive management, particularly the CEO, is vital in building a strong foundation for a health program. The steering committee should determine how much senior management support the program should expect, especially in the areas of budget and scope of activities provided. Numerous studies and testimonials will attest to the effectiveness of health management programs; collecting and presenting this information to senior management is a good first step in achieving buy-in from the senior level, and you can use it to establish program performance.

In addition to executive management, the support of other managers will be crucial to the health management program's success. Employees look to their supervisors for leadership, and managers can play a valuable and supportive role for subordinates. They can provide flexible time for participation, help to promote the programs, help to create a supportive culture, and support policies that are conducive to maintaining good health. Supervisors can be trained to understand and effectively support the program. In this capacity, they can be taught to recognize any emerging physical and/or mental health problems that may arise in their work force and provide encouragement and referrals.

The steering committee should get commitments from various departments that will be responsible for overseeing or delivering components of the program. If a department will be short-staffed because of the new program responsibilities, additional staff may need to be reassigned or hired.

A final step in determining employee support is to assess initial employee interest in a health management program. Administering employee interest surveys, which can be taken on the company Web site, is a good way to gauge interest. Surveys will help you learn about the programs in which the work force is interested, the media through which they are willing to participate, concerns they might have about things such as confidentiality and program quality, and the times and places in which they are willing to participate. Surveys are also a good first step in generating excitement and demonstrating that the program is about to become a reality.

Create a Vision

An overarching vision will give your program the direction and foundation it needs. By adopting a long-range vision, employees will be more inclined to accept healthy behavior as part of their work culture, instead of seeing it as an extraneous activity. If possible, you should create your program's mission statement to be consistent with and supportive of the company's mission. You can underscore in your health management program the values, ideals, and standards that drive your company, reminding employees of the company's reasons for doing business. Incorporating the health management program into the company vision and policy manual will give it credibility, as well as demonstrate that the company is committed to the long-term health and well-being of its workers.

The goals that you create in the beginning may well determine how quickly and effectively a health management program becomes productive. When setting goals, keep the end in mind, but remain flexible. What do you want your program to achieve in the first year? By the second and third years? It's important to set goals that are specific in nature; however, it is equally important to keep them flexible and appealing to end-users. If employees expect the health management program to be a "goal-driven burden," they are less likely to embrace it and participate. It is also important to avoid overwhelming employees by rolling out the program in a way that is easy to absorb during the first year. You may want to consider first-year goals that are more participation-focused and later-year goals that address risk reduction, disease stabilization, reduction in healthcare utilization, and financial impact. It is possible to have a health initiative that engages employees in ways they find appealing, while still maintaining a program that is evidence-based.

The objectives you set will help you achieve your goals. Objectives are most effective if they are set for both short-term and long-term achievements. Each goal can be broken into incremental objectives and placed on a timeline, until the goal is achieved. For instance, getting an 85% participation rate will involve communicating with employees effectively, offering incentives, scheduling follow-ups, and so forth.

When setting the program's goals and objectives remember that most programs focus on two primary goals:

- Keeping low-risk people at low risk

- Helping people with advanced risk factors, or who already have chronic illnesses, to improve their current conditions by improving or eliminating risk factors and controlling the diseases

The approach used to do this is often referred to as primary, secondary, and tertiary prevention, with primary prevention focused on keeping low-risk people at low risk, secondary prevention focused on controllable risk factors and behaviors, and tertiary prevention focused on stabilizing chronic illnesses. By keeping low-risk people at their low-risk status, and identifying individuals with multiple risk factors or chronic illnesses early, you can make efforts to avoid unnecessary medical interventions, such as emergency room visits, overnight hospital stays, and specific costly procedures, while increasing the well-being and productivity of the work force.

Setting and tracking goals and objectives will help to ensure that the program stays on course and that it produces measurable results in both health and financial terms over time.

Determine Realistic Staff and Budget Resources

Providing a sufficient budget for your health management program, to support staff and other fiscal needs, is crucial to its success. Comparative to the cost of healthcare, most programs don't need enormous resources to get off the ground. A health management initiative that is starved of vital assets, particularly financial assets, will have a difficult time succeeding in the company and may eventually wither from neglect.

A combination of internal staff members and external resources is often the most effective approach in launching and operating your health management initiative. To begin, the steering committee should determine the additional personnel, program advertising, program materials, IT support, and vendor costs that are needed for a successful program launch. To do this, it is necessary to project anticipated program utilization. Often, you can base these projections on your experience with similar programs, the experience of any consultants you are using, the experience of your potential vendors, and the advanced internal surveys and external research that the committee performed.

Total program cost is often expressed in terms of cost per employee per year. To determine this, forecast the total program cost for the start-up year and subsequent years, and then parse total costs out on a per-employee basis. In other words, add all anticipated costs and divide by the number of employees to determine cost per employee per year. It is not uncommon for this cost to be $150 to $200 per employee per year (not including incentive costs), but this varies widely based on program scope and company size. Smaller companies have fewer employees over which to spread fixed costs, often making their per-employee per-year cost higher than that of larger companies.

To determine whether existing staff members can handle the new responsibilities and demands of a health management program, or whether you will have to add additional staff members, you must ask several important questions. They are:

- What desired skill set is needed for effective delivery of the health management program? Does it currently exist within the company?

- If yes, does the internal staff have the time and resources to deliver the program? If the resources exist, but not the time, can staff members be added?

- If using existing internal resources, how will the new responsibilities be assigned to ensure quality execution?

- Does expertise and resources in the form of contractors exist within the community or at least the industry?

- Would the business case be easier to make for exclusive internal or external resources/ staffing or a combination of each?

Hire Additional Staff Members, Consultants, and Outside Vendors

If you determine that additional staff members or outside consultants are needed to deliver the health management program, hiring those people early in the planning process will help to ensure an effective launch and ongoing operation. You can later bring on any additional staff members as the need arises. Most successful health management programs have one person who is ultimately responsible for day-to-day operations. Having this individual visible as the leader of the program from the start lends legitimacy to the program, while giving employees a person or a department to go to for questions or clarifications.

Depending on the company's size and the program's scope, managing the overall health management initiative may be a full-time job. Internal staff members may be supplemented using outside vendors. Well-established and credible vendors have significant experience in health management programming. Partnering with them can bring significant expertise to the initiative, saving time and money and maximizing the chances of success. Further, these vendors specialize in the services they provide, so you benefit from their work with other clients. They are also insured for the services they provide, furnish a firewall of confidentiality between internal program leadership and employee participants, and are often less expensive than building internal resources, because they spread the overhead across their entire client base.

In some cases, community service groups such as the American Heart Association, the American Cancer Society, the American Diabetes Association, and the American Lung Association can provide additional resources. You also can tap other resources, such as nearby universities, local medical professionals, and public health departments. Your own health plans may also offer services that can help to supplement the program.

Create a Realistic Timeline

Launching a successful health management program often takes the better part of a year, although you can complete a launch in less time if some basic program elements are already in place. It is best when you time your launch to coincide with the benefit year. For most companies, this is either

fall or the first of the calendar year, though some have different benefit years. Although it is best to not time your launch to compete with other company events, such as product launches, national holidays, or other seasonal busy times, launching at or around benefit open enrollment can often give the program credibility, while piggybacking on other benefits communication. This will also establish the relationship between health management and benefit costs. In any event, superior program communication is essential.

Timelines, like goals, are most effective when they are recorded. Creating a schedule of critical dates and times may mean the difference between a focused and successful launch and a chaotic one. A detailed timeline is essential for those implementing the program.

Essential milestone dates, effectively communicated to potential participants, keeps the program in their minds' eye, helps them become mentally prepared for the program, makes the launch tangible, and sets their participation in the program in motion. A detailed timeline will also help to keep the components of the program that are related to each other in the proper sequence.

For instance, employees will need to complete HRAs before they participate in coaching, thus, the HRAs must be delivered first. Ultimately, a well-planned and well-executed timeline will keep the program on track, avoid duplication of effort, and result in a cost-efficient delivery. To establish your timeline, break down each component part of the program (communications, staffing, vendor selection, assessments, Web implementation, coaching, data collection, etc.) and the subcomponents for each, and estimate how long each will take to complete. Although many parts of the program will be ongoing, some items will need to be completed within a finite amount of time. With proper planning, the program can move forward without lag time.

Decide on and Develop Your Program's Rewards and Incentives

Motivating workers to make lifestyle changes can be a considerable undertaking. And it's no secret that many people respond better to carrots than sticks. Using both can be very effective.

According to a 2004 study by the SITE Foundation that was sponsored by the International Society for Performance Improvement, incentive programs increase performance an average of 22%. In fact, the study found that a 25% to 44% increase in performance was possible, if the incentive program was developed so as to balance the widest range of performance and motivational factors. The bottom line? Most companies that implement incentive programs as part of an overall health initiative will see better participation and health impact results than those that do not. The question

that lingers is whether these incentives are worth the cost when measuring return on investment.

Your incentive program must clearly communicate what employees and dependents must accomplish to be rewarded. It's a good idea to try to measure both qualitative and quantitative factors and to make sure they are fair and achievable for everyone in the company. If employees feel the incentives are not achievable or fair, they may give up on the entire program.

The kinds of incentives and awards you provide are important. Employees will more enthusiastically pursue rewards that are intrinsically important to them, and although cash is always of significant interest, other rewards can equally excite participants, without some of the drawbacks of money. For instance, incentives that are tied to the benefit plan can mobilize workers and their dependents to participate and improve their health, while drawing the connections between the cost of healthcare and lifestyle behavior. The most common method of using benefits-related incentives is to provide a personal premium reduction for people who participate in an annual HRA and biometric screening with additional incentives for a following-through with appropriate incentives. Placing money in health savings accounts on behalf of the employee is another way employees can be rewarded through the benefit plan. In some cases, the benefit plan itself can provide incentives that help employees become good purchasers of effective healthcare services by paying for preventive services at higher rates than restorative care, and encouraging good consumerism.

In addition to money and benefits-related incentives, some programs still provide merchandise or other types of gifts. Some vendors and stand-alone incentive companies specialize in providing a host of ready-made merchandise to organizations to use as incentives. Many of these companies have catalogs of appropriate gifts and will handle ordering, fulfillment, and emblazing company logos.

Promote the Program throughout the Company

Proper introduction to and ongoing communication of your health management program is vital to its success. Your employees must recognize the health management effort and value its importance.

Your program should start with a comprehensive marketing and promotion plan that will be aimed at all organization levels and that recognizes the organization's different constituencies. Buy-in from all of these groups will be necessary for a successful program. If you want consumers to engage, health management programming must be

effectively sold to workers and their dependents. Effective communication will maximize the chances that they will hear, understand, and, most important, act on the message.

One option you may want to consider is having an outside firm develop the program's communication plan. Public relations firms, some health programming consulting groups, and many service vendors can provide this service effectively. The outsourcing of plan development could save staff time, help to keep the program on schedule, and recruit expertise that may not exist in-house.

Promoting the program message must become the rule for employees, not the exception. One way to achieve this is the ongoing use of existing company communications to promote the health management program, such as in-house newsletters, benefits communications, safety communiqués, and broadcast e-mails and voice mails. A well-planned effort that continually utilizes these resources can be both effective and cost-efficient.

Additionally, having an endorsement from the company CEO or other senior executive will lend the program credibility. As a result, a quarterly update to senior managers on progress, new programs, and other pertinent information can keep the program top of mind for employees.

Implement the Program

Once you have most of the program's components planned, it is time to launch the program. This is best achieved by a phased-in approach, so as not to overwhelm the program's end-users and so that effective implementation can occur with the resources available. We have devoted Chapter 6 to a discussion on implementing your health management program.

The program should be designed to allow participants to have early success. Access to online tools, easy enrollment in programs, and participation in HRAs and biometric screenings are all good places to start.

Issuing a letter from the CEO or president announcing the launch of the program to every employee will underscore its importance and help establish a culture of health throughout the organization. Recognizing the value that senior management places on the program may also induce more employee participation.

Make sure everyone in the organization knows the program's leaders and understands how the program works. As the launch occurs, encourage feedback from all levels of the organization. As the program progresses, try to make incremental changes according to the feedback, until the program becomes efficient and integrated into the company culture. Although this may take time, these small achievements can yield huge rewards.

Make Ongoing Evaluation a Priority

The ongoing evaluation of your health management program is perhaps one of the most important efforts you will undertake. As the program launches and while it continues, collect and evaluate data. Also collect participant satisfaction and anecdotal information. The steering committee should be responsible for establishing a plan for how to gather information, warehouse it, evaluate it, and report on it. We will talk more about measurement and evaluation in Chapter 8. For now, consider the following evaluation questions:

- How many employees used the program? Specifically, who used the program?

- What are the overall perceptions of the program's effectiveness?

- What is the level of participant satisfaction with the program?

- Did participants continue with the program or stop using it over time?

- Were some activities and events more popular or effective? Which ones, and why?

- Has the culture of health improved within the organization?

- Do employees feel that the information in the program is easy to use and understand?

- Can employees easily access the online tools provided?

- Are employees satisfied with the incentives and rewards offered? Do the incentives drive participation and health improvement?

- Do employees feel that their privacy is secure?

- Has there been a net reduction in the amount of risk in the population?

- Are persons with chronic illnesses more stable on average because of the program? Has there been measurable clinical improvement?

- What has been the program's economic impact?

It will also be important to determine whether the company's initial goals and objectives are being met. If not, programmatic adjustments will be necessary. If goals and objectives were met, recalibrating the target and taking the program to new heights should be the course of action.

Modify or Change the Program

Once you evaluate the data collected and answer some of these questions, you may decide that your health management program needs adjustment. Phasing in changes will make them less disruptive and more effective.

Each chapter of this book will provide information that will be helpful in both the original development of your health management initiative and its ongoing operation. We will detail areas that you need to consider and implement to create an effective program. We will devote Chapter 9 to breathing new life into an existing health management program that may have lost its momentum. Taken as a whole, each chapter can help you make the large or small changes needed to develop the kind of health management initiative that will meet the needs of employees and dependents and help you achieve your organizational goals and objectives.

Keep in mind that by personally involving employees in the management of their own health and in controlling the costs associated with disease, you can more effectively impact the overall health and productivity of your work force and control spiraling healthcare costs. Conceived and delivered effectively, your health management program can become a valuable and strategic business tool.

Chapter 3

The Importance of
Tailoring Programs

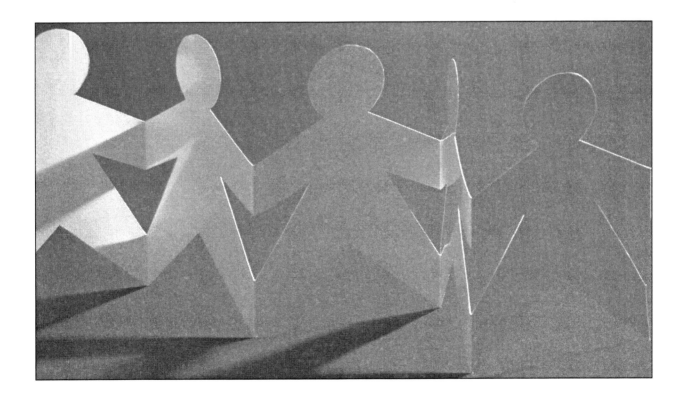

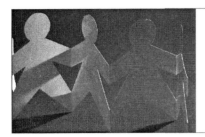

The Importance of Tailoring Programs

A health management program is only as successful as its participants, so the importance of enthusiastic employee buy-in cannot be stressed enough. Without endorsement and participation from most people in the organization, your health management program could stumble or wither from neglect. Tailoring specific programs and activities to achieve the benefits of good health, while also meeting your employees' needs and preferences, can ensure that your health management initiative will enjoy long-lasting success.

To maximize cost-efficiency and return on investment (ROI), you should utilize a multitiered program in which participants are triaged into programs based on risk level. Persons at the highest risk are provided the most aggressive care, whereas persons with less risk are provided less aggressive care.

The Health Impact Model

Figure 3.1 presents the recommended model. It provides a picture of the model, how participants flow through it annually based on health status, and how other support services are provided to maximize program success. In the figure are four major areas of emphasis.

These include:

- Engage and Incent

- Assess/Activate/Refer

- Educate/Motivate/Support

- Measurement and Reporting

We will explain each of these in detail.

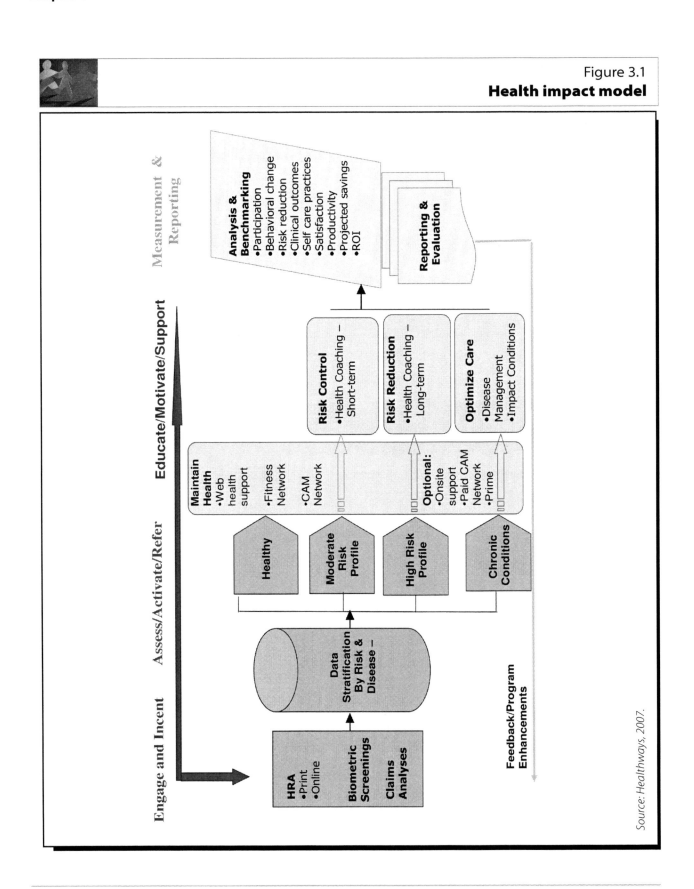

Figure 3.1
Health impact model

Source: Healthways, 2007.

Engage and Incent

Communication

Good communication of a health management initiative is essential in maximizing participation, trust, credibility, and ultimate program success. You must engage the target audience to encourage participation in early program elements, such as health risk assessments (HRAs) and biometric screenings, as well as in ongoing behavior change and disease management interventions. Engagement communications will continually advertise the program and should have four areas of focus:

- Informing

- Mobilizing

- Supporting follow-through

- Supporting a healthy culture on an ongoing basis

You should approach program communications with the same rigor that a manufacturer would use in launching a new product. You must help the potential market to understand the value of the health management program, what is in it for them, and how and when they can access it. You must also encourage this audience to continue participating in the health management programs and remind them of their value. The engagement communications should come in many forms of media (e-mails, bulletin boards, company news-letters, home mailings, etc.). To maximize the value, you should develop and carry out a detailed communications plan. You should design the plan to reach people who use different media, have varying interests, are at different stages of readiness, and are demographically and culturally diverse. Advertising agencies, consulting firms, service vendors, and communications firms can provide assistance in creating a dynamic communications plan.

Incentives

In many cases, employees need external motivation until the value of health improvement becomes internalized. Incentives can motivate employees and their dependents to participate and change, and can be an important success factor for your health management program. Providing incentives for participation, health improvement, or both, demonstrates the importance your organization places on healthy behavior and makes a strong statement that your culture supports healthy practices. Depending on the nature of the incentive, incentive programs can also help participants become more informed about the company benefit plans, how to become good healthcare consumers, and the link between their behavior and health-related costs to both them and the company.

The use of incentives in health management, especially in primary and secondary prevention, is not new. What is new is the prevalence of the use of incentives and the creative approaches being taken. Today, incentives are usually of higher value than they were in the past, they are often attached to benefits, and in most companies with wellness programs, they are the rule rather than the exception. They are also more structured. For instance, many incentive plans have several tiers. There is some amount of reward for being assessed through an HRA or biometric screening, some amount of reward for participating in a risk-appropriate intervention, and some amount of reward provided for successfully completing the intervention. Incentives often include:

- Reductions in personal benefit premiums

- Money provided in a health savings account

- Gift cards

- Merchandise

- Cash (with cash there are often personal tax ramifications for the participant)

You will also want to determine what activities, behaviors, or outcomes you wish to reward. Some possibilities include:

- HRA participation and/or biometric screening participation

- Intervention participation

- Intervention completion

- Certain behaviors (e.g., good nutrition, physical activity, not smoking, etc.)

- Certain health outcomes (e.g., blood pressure, cholesterol, body mass index [BMI], etc.)

In terms of incentive value, a rule of thumb is $200 per employee. However, you may have to take other factors into account, such as the average pay of the work force, the company culture, the time between action and receipt of the incentive, and the perceived value of the incentive. We have seen effective incentive values range from a $2 cafeteria voucher to $2,000 in benefit cost reductions, depending on the circumstances. We have also seen programs that have been highly successful without incentives, and programs in which the incentive brought only marginal improvements while significantly increasing program cost, thereby negatively impacting the program ROI. Thus, choosing to use incentives and deciding on the nature of those incentives is important when developing a health management program.

Depending on how incentive programs are structured and positioned, they can provide a carrot, a stick, or both. For instance, providing a reduction in the personal health benefit premium for nonsmokers feels like a carrot to the nonsmokers, but like a stick to smokers, even if the incentive is intended to be a carrot to encourage people not to smoke. Although carrots tend to be better received in most cultures, the use of the stick is becoming more common. As healthcare costs continue to rise, it is likely that use of the stick will continue to increase as well.

The keys for a successful incentive program include keeping it simple, effectively communicating it to end-users, building trust through efficient administration, and keeping participants informed. To this end, implementing an incentive program raises questions that you need to address within the company:

- What are the incentives?

- What is the value of each incentive?

- How should you structure and administer the incentive?

- What are the legal ramifications of incentive programs?

We will be addressing some of these questions throughout the book, but it is important to think about them and the answers needed within the context of your own company culture. Incentives are becoming customary in wellness programs, and in some cases they are associated with outcomes, especially if they are administered by health plans. It is likely incentives will continue to evolve and become more strategic in nature.

Administering incentives can be complex and difficult if you do not set up the incentives

properly in the beginning. A lack of preparation and forethought can negatively impact employee enthusiasm and participation. And because most incentive programs depend heavily on information technology for both tracking and rewarding recipients, putting electronic mechanisms in place to keep participants informed is crucial. Involving the IT department early in program development improves your chances of success in setting up and administering the incentive program.

In administering incentives, you must be careful to award them fairly. You must set business and policy rules for new hires, late entrants, and employee challenges to the program. To make administration easier, try to avoid complex incentive programs, ones that are too difficult to communicate or fulfill. Further, having a way for participants to confirm that incentives have been awarded, such as a Web site on which they can check status, will reduce the administrative burden of addressing inquiries. One caution is to make sure the structure does not inadvertently breach confidentiality.

For instance, if an incentive can be gained by participating in a variety of health management programs regardless of health status, and incentive administrators within your organization learn only who has received an incentive award, there is no breach. However, if a list were to be circulated that indicated who was rewarded for participating in the disease management program that would be a breach because it exposes the people on the list as having a chronic illness.

There are other complicating factors as well. Some incentive programs require participants to meet certain health standards, such as being at a normal blood pressure, having a BMI below a certain level, having a cholesterol level in a normal range, and so on. In cases where health status is a consideration for incentives, the Health Insurance Portability and Accountability Act of 1996 sets specific standards about what can and can't be done. In general, the size of the award must be limited, the incentive must be designed to promote health or prevent disease, there must be an annual qualification opportunity, the program must be provided to all similarly situated individuals, and potential participants must be notified that accommodations will be provided for those who would be unable to participate due to some form of impairment or hardship. In addition, a number of other state and federal laws can apply in some cases, so legal review before setting up an incentive program is always prudent. See Chapter 7 for more information on legal ramifications.

Another point of leverage for incentive programs is to bring in providers. Many health plans drive to new levels of provider engagement through pay-for-performance (P4P) programs. Such programs incent providers, most often physicians, to focus on certain key aspects of care that the health plan seeks to improve.

An opportunity exists for employers to direct their health plans to align provider P4P programs with member incentive programs. The point, therefore, is to focus on creating a logical synergy and partnership between doctor and patient to work together toward common health and wellness goals. This is strategic alignment at its best.

Studies have found that incentives drive participation, participation drives health improvement, and health improvement drives healthcare costs and productivity improvement. With this in mind, it is important to offer incentives that are of perceived value to employees, while maintaining a sensible and cost-effective approach for the company.

When creating incentive programs, keep in mind that you don't want to set the bar too high or make the incentive too lucrative. This may only induce cheating and unnecessary payouts, with the point of health improvement lost in the message.

By paying careful attention to the kinds of incentives you implement, you can ensure that potential participants will enthusiastically receive and support your health management initiative. Having employees physically and mentally buy in to the program and embrace a new healthy culture within the company will make the implementation of new policies and initiatives much easier.

Assess, Activate, and Refer

Once you have mobilized employees through engagement and incentives, a first step in the delivery of the Health Impact Model is to assess each person who is eligible to participate. HRAs, biometric screenings, and claims analyses are commonly used for this purpose.

Health risk assessments and biometric screenings

An HRA and biometric screening provides the baseline and starting point of a health management initiative and should be considered the first crucial step in drawing participants into the program. Conducting these initiatives through a combination of Web, paper, and on-site programming allows a significant part of your employee population to receive HRA and screenings cost-efficiently, especially if an incentive is used. HRAs and screenings allow employees to benchmark their health when their status results are aggregated. They also provide the means for the organization to target programs, continuously improving the quality for the programs and the outcomes. Based on these results, you can focus your health management programming on the specific needs of employees and the organization, and position it for maximum impact.

It is recommended that you introduce an online HRA that has a paper/pencil alternative, and that you provide on-site screenings to employees and dependents so they may receive a comprehensive health assessment. The on-site screenings also allow you to collect objective biometric data. This is important because many employees and dependents don't know their cholesterol, blood pressure, and other biometric indicators or in some cases are not honest about them.

Having both employees and their spouses in the program together is advantageous because they can provide each other mutual support, and often, the health-related cost of the spouse is higher than that of the employee. Providing access to the HRA online can significantly reduce the cost while effectively reaching both the spouse and employee. New employees should be offered HRAs and biometric screenings as part of their orientation.

Claims analysis

Claims analysis will also be used to identify persons eligible for disease management and, in some cases, health coaching (e.g., obesity codes, metabolic syndrome codes, etc.). Although not all employees take an HRA or screening, all employees who seek medical care file claims, so this information can be highly valuable in better understanding a greater percentage of your overall population's needs.

Activate and refer

Once HRA, biometric screening, and claims information is known, you should be prepared to activate and refer the population into an appropriate intervention. You can use the assessment data to stratify the population into the following four primary groups:

- Healthy

- Moderate-risk profile

- High-risk profile

- Chronic conditions

Participants may be activated based on their health and risk status. All participants should be provided with services to help them stay healthy. People with risk factors or chronic conditions should be further referred to interventions that help them control or reduce risk or optimize chronic-disease care.

By taking this step, you can conduct your interventions strategically, maximizing the intervention cost-efficiency and potential for health impact, both of which are important in generating the best ROI. Figure 3.2 shows how the population usually is stratified on average.

Figure 3.2
Hierarchy of morbidity

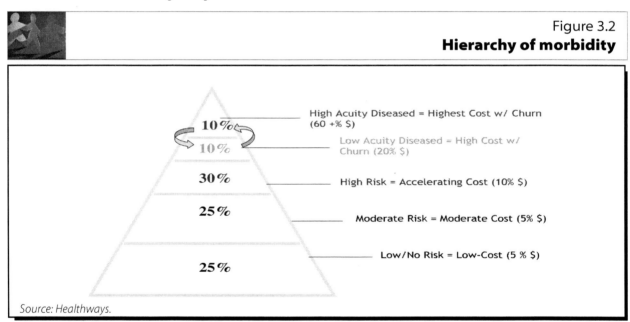

Source: Healthways.

Interventions to Educate, Motivate, and Support

The Educate, Motivate, and Support interventions shown in Figure 3.1 are designed to maintain healthy behaviors, control or reduce risk factors, and/or optimize the care of people with chronic conditions.

Behavior change is a key component of all health management programs, and applying the latest in the behavioral sciences will enhance the efficacy of this component. Over the years, the Transtheoretical Model of Change, a theoretical model of behavior change that has been the basis for developing successful interventions to promote changes in health behavior, has dramatically changed the way behavior change programs are developed and delivered. You can use these different strategies depending on the participant's level of readiness to make any given behavior change. Additionally, adult education research reveals that adults learn best when:

- They can choose from a variety of learning strategies

- The materials or sessions are interactive

- They can see results or demonstrate their learning immediately and in a real-world setting

- They receive support from family and friends

- They can address pros and cons to change (decisional balance)

The "Maintain Health" programs that are delivered as part of the Health Impact Model are available to all people, regardless of their health status. Although these may differ among organizations, many programs are commonly used.

Health maintenance

One of the most important efforts that you should undertake in delivering an employee health management effort is to keep the healthy people from developing risk factors or chronic illnesses. Thus, providing programs that support healthy people in their efforts is essential. Programs of this nature need not be expensive, and they are often called "pull" programs because the healthy people will be drawn to them. Examples of pull programs include Web-based exercise and nutrition trackers, fitness center networks, availability of complementary and alternative-medicine providers, and awareness information. The old adage about these types of programs was "if you provide them, only the healthy people will use them," stated as though that were a problem. The new adage is "the more healthy people we can get to use these kinds of services, the better." A growing body of evidence demonstrates that it is less expensive to keep someone healthy than it is to fix him or her once he or she develops risk factors or a chronic illness. Although pull programs may target the healthy, they can benefit people at any state of health.

In the following sections, we describe some programs designed to maintain health.

Physical activity

Increased physical activity has been demonstrated to improve health, motivate participants to make other appropriate lifestyle changes, and create a positive ROI. By including specific, fun, and useful physical activities in your health management program, you will increase the odds that employees will join and stay interested. Elements of a specific physical activity initiative may include the following:

- Special action plans implemented to promote pedometer use and to encourage employees and their dependents to log 10,000 steps per day. Complementary pedometers will help to support better enrollment.

- Online curricula concerning physical activity, including programs to help participants develop and track proper fitness.

- Support communities where exercisers can find each other via the Web or in person to share ideas or arrange "buddy" workouts.

- Walking routes around work locations that are mapped and recorded.

- Discount rates with local fitness centers or participation in a discount or paid fitness network.

- Various exercise clubs (e.g., walking, running, bicycling, etc.).

- Discounts on home exercise equipment.

- A community resources listing of fitness centers and services.

- Encouragement of stairway use.

- Use of nearby walking trails, if available.

Figure 3.3
The many benefits of lifestyle change

New Value Proposition

Exercise →

Benefits of exercise

- Reduce risk for Heart Disease and Stroke

- Back Pain

- Osteoporosis

- Psychological benefits including stress hardiness

- A minimum of at least 30 minutes of moderate intensity exercise daily resulted in a reduced risk of coronary heart disease by more than 2-fold (*Diabetes Care, 2005*)
- Walking and losing 15 pounds decreased the risk of getting diabetes by 58% (*NIH Study; n=3,284*)

Source: Healthways.

Stress management

People reporting high stress statistically have higher annual healthcare expenditures than people with any other singular risk factor. Because of its relationship to depression and other mental health disorders, stress is of considerable concern from both a healthcare cost and a productivity perspective. The good news is that stress can be mitigated; resulting in happier, more productive employees while creating opportunities for cost savings. To help your workers manage stress, you should implement programs such as the following:

- Online stress management resources that address the topic broadly and provide tools for better controlling life events

- Support communities that people dealing with particular types of stressors can be a part of via the Web or in person

- Focused programming for areas or occupations where the HRA indicated greatest concerns

- Efforts to educate employees on stress-related topics, such as resiliency, problem-solving skill development, influencing skill development, and violence prevention

- Stress management and awareness integrated into manager training programs

- Stress management included in orientation/ supervisor training

Weight maintenance/reduction and nutrition

Obesity and being overweight have been directly associated with many diseases, including heart disease, diabetes, musculoskeletal injury, and cancers. Obesity often results from poor nutrition and lack of physical activity, making it treatable. Particularly for older workers, being overweight has been correlated with significantly higher healthcare costs. Wellness efforts to control weight and obesity will have a positive impact on individuals and worker productivity, but also will have an impact on healthcare costs.

Figure 3.4
Obesity facts

Obesity is not an isolated condition— associated with:

- ✔ Type 2 diabetes

- ✔ Cardiovascular disease

- ✔ Cancer (endometrial, postmenopausal breast, kidney, colon)

- ✔ Musculoskeletal disorders

- ✔ Sleep apnea

- ✔ Gallbladder disease

Statistics indicate that more than 65% of Americans are overweight or obese. A state-of-the-art weight management and nutrition effort should be one of the cornerstones of your health management program. Implementing such a program can help to control weight and improve eating habits. Studies have shown that people lose more weight and keep it off longer if they are part of a structured program, rather than trying to go it alone. An effective weight management program might include the following:

- One-on-one assistance through coaching and other personal attention

- One-on-one and group counseling by dietitians

- Weight management and nutrition classes

- Online weight control and nutrition support programs

- Support communities where people working to eat nutritiously or to lose weight can take part via the Web or in person

- Assistance for people with diseases which are related to obesity (e.g., diabetes)

- Weight reduction/maintenance challenges among departments

- Changes in vending machine and cafeteria selections to support improved eating and weight loss in the company culture

- Integration of physical activity efforts with weight loss efforts

- Community programs such as Weight Watchers

- Ongoing communications in company and program media highlighting the importance of proper eating and weight control

Figure 3.5
Cost of obesity

Total cost to U.S. companies is estimated at $13 billion per year[1]

- Health insurance costs $8 billion
- Paid sick leave $2.4 billion
- Life insurance $1.8 billion
- Disability insurance $1 billion

Obese individuals have higher health care utilization rates[2]

- 36% higher inpatient and outpatient spending
- 77% higher medication spending
- 45% more inpatient days
- 48% more expenditures over $5,000
- 11% higher annual health care costs

[1] *Prevention Makes Common Cents: Estimated Economic Costs of Obesity to U.S. Business, DHHS*
[2] *Health Risks and Behavior: The Impact on Medicala Costs, Control Data Corporation, 1987*

Tobacco control

Tobacco use is one of the leading killers of Americans and is responsible for significant health-related costs. In spite of this, more than 20% of Americans still smoke. Therefore, it is essential to implement a best-practice tobacco cessation program as part of your overall health management program. Tobacco cessation efforts have significantly reduced the number of Americans who smoke, demonstrating that such programs can be successful. Tobacco cessation is of particular importance for older workers, as they face the highest risks of morbidity, mortality, and high healthcare costs from the use of tobacco.

Because tobacco use can result in significant insurance costs for a company, it must be addressed. And it's no secret that many people try to quit smoking every year. Having an effective tobacco cessation program in place will allow employees the opportunity to quit, as well as encourage them to engage in other parts of the program that will help them maintain weight and control stress while quitting. Best-practice programs utilize personalized attention and nicotine replacement therapies to most effectively help people quit. A good smoking cessation effort will include elements such as:

- Online curricula and telephone support

- Support communities that people can be a part of via the Web or in person

- Acupuncture and other alternative therapy discounts

- Environmental changes, such as eliminating smoking areas

- An aggressive smoking policy

- A benefits "penalty" for smokers

- Benefits coverage for nicotine replacement therapy and tobacco cessation drugs

Pregnancy education

The cost of a complicated pregnancy can be astronomical. Research shows that simply avoiding tobacco and alcohol and utilizing proper nutrition during pregnancy can result in a healthier mother and baby and a normal-cost delivery. Education on other prenatal factors can also provide value. For these reasons, you should consider a pregnancy education initiative to be a part of your health management program. Such an initiative highlights company support for workers and their families. If possible, you should include additional wellness professionals (dietitians, health coaches, etc.) in your company's pregnancy education efforts. Pregnancy education is of even greater value in young work forces.

Self-care

Medical self-care, one of the original health management strategies, has been shown to generate relatively immediate health improvements and cost savings. Because of this, self-care should be a prominent component of your health management program. By utilizing a comprehensive yet efficient approach to self-care, your program will have the potential to eliminate unnecessary expenditures and to direct the care that is provided to the most cost-effective and medically-effective venue.

The self-care program should encourage employees and spouses to practice judicious self-care and become efficient healthcare consumers. By eliminating unnecessary physician's office and emergency room visits, a company can expect to lower its overall healthcare costs. Further, by helping employees and dependents better recognize emergent health events, you can ensure that they can get to the most effective treatment venues more quickly. You can implement self-care strategies through newsletters, hard-copy manuals distributed to each employee, nurse lines, or online services. A combination of these has proven to be most effective.

Complementary and alternative healthcare

You can give employees and dependents access to complementary and alternative healthcare through either affinity discounts or fully paid programs. Often, these lower cost programs can greatly assist employees and dependents in their efforts to stay healthy. Specialties might include acupuncture, massage, Pilates, personal trainers, yoga instructors, and chiropractors. Participants often take

their own pathway to remaining healthy, and complementary and alternative healthcare can be part of their support network.

Moderate-risk, high-risk, and chronically ill participants

Lifestyle behaviors and chronic diseases account for more than 50% of healthcare usage by employees. By addressing risk factors and nonchronic or acute conditions early, you can avoid chronic illness and its associate costs to the organization.

Many people with health risks or chronic diseases fail to take action on their own behalf. Moreover, these people (especially those who already have chronic illnesses) tend to be significantly more costly in terms of healthcare outlays, particularly in terms of medical interventions and prescription drugs. These people are also the ones most ensconced in their present behavior, and thus are the hardest to change. Therefore, individualized efforts aimed at specific employees and dependents are often necessary to have an impact in behavior change. Although usually more expensive, these programs often generate a significant ROI because they have both a high-cost impact potential and a track record of success. What's more, because of the effectiveness of these programs, employees are able to see greater personal results, and thus can stay more engaged with them.

Health coaching

Using health coaching for persons with multiple risk factors can help to avoid future healthcare costs by preventing a portion of the population from developing a chronic disease or serious health condition. Thus, health coaching is a cost avoidance strategy. Health coaching is often offered to employees and dependents who demonstrate elevated health risks on their HRA, biometric screenings, or claims data. They can be offered a lower-intensity health coaching program to people with moderate risk factors and a higher-intensity program to people with higher or multiple risk factors. Program intensity is usually defined by the number of contacts, length of contacts, number of months in the program, and similar factors.

Health coaching is usually delivered by phone, by e-mail, or in person. In most cases, coaching involves a person-to-person interaction; however, Web-based tools have been developed with artificial intelligence to simulate the coaching experience. Risks most often addressed through health coaching include behaviorial factors, such as nutrition, stress, smoking, and physical activity, and biometric factors such as cholesterol, blood sugar, blood pressure, and weight.

Disease management

To be most effective, your health management initiative should have a disease management component that focuses on clinical improvement, healthy-behavior improvement, self-care behaviors,

appropriate surveillance care, and other practices necessary for self-control of specific diseases. This will aid in the management of important clinical indicators, while underscoring the value your company places on healthy employees. You should offer a disease management program to all employees identified as having a targeted disease through the analysis of claims, HRAs, or screening data, or who demonstrate a willingness to be part of such a program through self-referral.

Some of the diseases that you should consider for the disease management program include coronary artery disease, heart failure, diabetes, asthma, hypertension, and depression. Other diseases impact employee productivity and generate cost, although they are not often catastrophic. These impact conditions should be effectively managed to maximize the value of the disease management effort. Some of these conditions include sleep disturbance disorders/fatigue, allergic rhinitis, stress management, responsible drinking, migraine (marginal), atrial fibrillation, low back pain, osteoarthritis, fibromyalgia, and osteoporosis.

Offering these disease management programs can effectively control employees' disease conditions, helping them avoid unnecessary medical interventions such as emergency room visits, overnight hospital stays, and specific costly procedures. Disease management is most often delivered by phone, but other media, such as home monitoring, automated calling, and Web-based programs, are becoming more prevalent. A combination of all of these resources is usually most effective.

Since the proverbial 20% of employees spend 80% of the healthcare dollars, and a majority of employees and their dependents often exhibit a risk profile showing a high potential to eventually progress to a costly disease state, disease management and health coaching programs that reach this group can help to avert future disease, resulting in early and immediate cost reductions.

In fact, in many cases, minimal effort can result in significant cost savings potential, which is why it is so critical for all employees to become enthusiastic users of disease management and health coaching programs if they are eligible.

Measurement and Reporting

Measurement and reporting is an essential part of the Health Impact Model. Factors that are often measured and reported include:

- Participation

- Behavioral change

- Risk reduction

- Clinical outcomes

- Self-management practice improvement

- Change in medicare care patterns

- Productivity improvement

- Satisfaction

- Projected savings

- ROI

The information that is collected is used to make sure the program is on target and to make mid-course adjustments. It is also used to determine the program's longitudinal health and cost impact. We will provide more information on measurement and evaluation later in the book.

Once the component parts of the Health Impact Model are in place, it is recommended that the program be communicated to all employees and dependents. We will talk more about communication later in the book

Chapter 4

The Tools and Technology

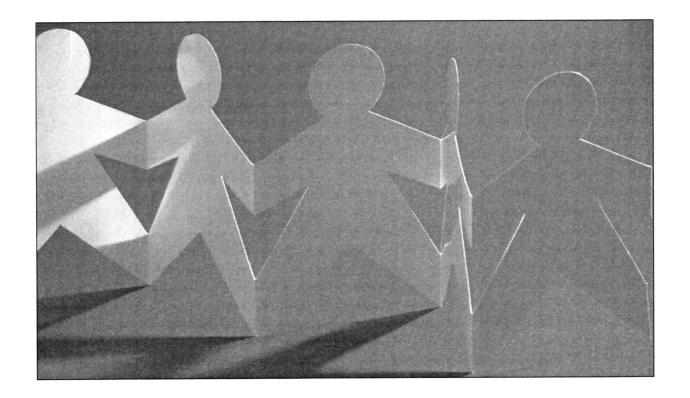

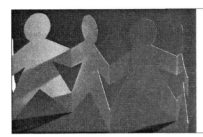

The Tools and Technology

Online and Technology Initiatives

As we have discussed thus far in this book, there are many ways to approach your health management program. Regardless of the programs and initiatives you include in your program, an arsenal of online technology coupled with real-life tools can create a potent formula for success. The importance of these tools is that they allow for enhanced engagement. It's a simple truth that you can't change a person's behavior if you never effectively reach him or her.

With these technologies and strategies in place, you will be able to implement ongoing behavior change programs that will have a significant impact on employees. Implemented and used successfully, the following online and personal intervention recommendations can persuade employees to make simple, day-to-day choices that can have lasting repercussions in their lives.

By creating easy-to-use online Internet interfaces, you enable your employees to register for programs, track their progress, vie for incentives, and communicate with other employees involved in the health management program. These online wellness and incentive initiatives will drive program participation, while creating support and enthusiasm for the program.

With a reported 75% of all U.S. households having Internet access at home, smart companies are presenting many of their health management initiatives online for 24-hour access. Online programs can be especially effective if your employees are spread throughout a large geographical area.

There is growing evidence that use of the computer and the Internet as a wellness partner is working. For instance, more than 50 successful online behavior change programs have been implemented at The Builders Association of Northern Nevada, Brigham Young University, and The Washoe County School District in Reno, NV.

The Health Risk Assessment

The health risk assessment (HRA) is at the corner-stone of many company wellness programs because of its ability to pinpoint and evaluate an employee's current health status. These electronic or hard-copy questionnaires gather important information about employee health, lifestyle, and risk factors.

Thanks to the proliferation of health management programs, a variety of HRA tools and vendors now exist. Most HRAs consist of 85 to 100 questions and are written around the eighth-grade level, so most employees can understand the questions. An HRA can take, on average, 20 minutes to complete, and usually asks about height, weight, blood pressure, cholesterol levels, smoking habits, lifestyle choices, diet and eating habits, and exercise regimes.

After completing the HRA, the employee receives a customized report, tailored to his or her health status and indicating any health-related risks. This report will be either mailed to the respondent within two weeks, or provided electronically if the employee answered questions online. HRAs are an excellent tool for demonstrating an employee's risk of diabetes, heart disease, asthma, or other chronic conditions.

Most respected HRAs cost between $5 and $15 per participant for the electronic version and $10 to $25 per participant for the hard-copy version, including mailing fees. Be aware that additional set-up fees and other initial account costs may be charged to the company when the HRA is launched. Make sure you ask your HRA vendor about any hidden or added fees you may incur.

Confidentiality is crucial to the success of the HRA. Without a complete assurance of confidentiality, employees will be reluctant to complete an HRA, and because much of your wellness program hinges on the HRA, you must remove this barrier. Employees should understand that the company will not have access to any of their health information in recognizable form. Although reports will be generated concerning overall statistics, make sure to emphasize that no individual health information pertaining to specific employees will be known or shared.

HRA incentives

The debate over what incentive to offer, if any, for completing an HRA continues. However, most agree that the HRA is the first step in getting employees interested in a wellness program and clarifying their current or possible future health risks and conditions. HRAs have the ability to get—and keep—an employee's attention because seeing evidence of the impact of their behaviors is hard to ignore. Without incentives, it is hard to get employees motivated to take action. Studies have shown that without incentives, participation in HRAs drops to 10% or less. However, with the right kinds of incentives, participation can soar to up 90% to 95%.

Incentives, which have already been discussed, can range from trinkets (T-shirts, mugs, etc.) to gym memberships, merchandise, gift certificates, cash incentives, and the lowering of insurance premiums. Remember that not all cultures require or even are accepting of incentives. Thus, while they can be valuable in driving HRA participation, they are not always necessary.

Communicating the availability of HRAs

It is crucial that you emphasize the importance of taking an HRA to each employee in your organization. Without an effective communications plan, chances are your employees will be less inclined to participate.

You should develop an overarching communications plan months in advance that defines an HRA, explains why it is important, and instructs employees how they can take it (either online or in paper form). Because of the sensitivity of HRAs, it is vitally important to communicate that the HRA process is conducted to support employees in their own efforts to live healthy lifestyles and that the organization cares about every workers' good health.

Make it clear that the HRA is a tool designed to help employees understand their health risks, and provides information on what they can do to minimize the risk of health problems. Also, make sure to emphasize the confidentiality of the tool in all communications.

One to two weeks before the HRA launch, post announcements in a variety of places, such as on the company's intranet site and in the company's in-house newsletter, on bulletin boards, and, if financially feasible, send a letter to each employee's home. These announcements should stress the constant message that the organization is interested in maintaining a healthy culture, and mobilize the participant to take action. Once again, the use of technology in the form of online communications can prove invaluable as it is inexpensive and reaches people efficiently.

Your HRA vendor should be able to assist you in setting up the HRA and provide advice on the best approach to communicate it to your work force.

For best results, you should plan to conduct your HRA every year. This will give you the opportunity to gather information longitudally, which will reveal yearly health trends in the data. It will also help employees keep track of their own health trends, on an ongoing basis, potentially motivating their continual action in maintaining good behavior.

Conducting a Health Culture Audit

In conjunction with the HRA, your company should consider conducting a companywide health culture audit. This audit is an instrument for measuring an organization's cultured support of health and productivity. What makes the health culture audit so valuable is the honest feedback received from your employees. The audit, if administered properly, can reveal individual and group perceptions regarding health and well-being related to the organization. This is important because of the enormous impact a company's culture has on an employee's mental and physical health. This audit will provide a baseline and important information on what needs to change across the organization to create an environment that is supportive to maintaining good health.

As an example, the Lifegain Health Culture Audit measures norms and values related to major wellness themes, such as self-responsibility, healthy fun, mutual respect, and achieving one's full potential. In addition, the survey examines peer support and organizational support systems that can make or break employee efforts to adopt healthier and more productive practices.

Each health culture audit also examines work climate factors, such as sense of community, shared vision, positive outlook, and health risk behaviors, including work-life balance and smoking. Survey questions can be added to assess program satisfaction, barriers to participation, and employee preferences regarding program content. The health culture audit even provides basic financial forecast tools designed to determine the economic impact of your efforts. Results can be reported by demographic and employment groups.

Wellness Teams

A wellness team can bring together people from throughout the organization who can represent others in the business. If properly set up, this team can help plan the program, suggest best ways to communicate, and will be its advocates. As such, a wellness team can be an important tool in assuring success.

According to Dr. David Hunnicutt, president of Wellness Council of America in Omaha, NE, there are ways to approach teams and team-building in health management programs that can aid success if undertaken properly. He recommends that team members be formally appointed by the CEO or other senior executives to serve the program. This formal appointment highlights the responsibility and strategic value the company places on the health management program, and clarifies the committee's roles and responsibilities when it comes to overseeing employee health.

This formal appointment also avoids the problem of depending on volunteers to steer the program, as these people may or may not be available to make the health management program a priority, especially if another pressing matter arises in the workplace. The appointment makes clear to everyone, particularly the appointee, that the health management program is important and the duties assigned need to be carried out.

To add authenticity and weight to the appointment, Hunnicutt recommends including health promotion responsibilities to the employee's job description. Today's workplaces can be hectic, with multiple priorities competing for attention. Writing health promotion duties into a job description can prevent those duties from falling by the wayside when more pressing matters clamor for attention. The employee doesn't have to devote all of his or her time to the health management program, but by including responsibility in the job description you can ensure that the employee and other workers understand that it is *part* of the job.

This approach can eliminate confusion regarding what needs to be done, while also helping an appointee justify time spent on a health management project. Without such support, volunteers may feel subtle pressure to drop their involvement to a low-priority category.

Hunnicutt suggests making employees across the organization aware of the wellness committee, its members, and its roles. This lends credence and credibility to the team and the programs as a whole. Because the company is appointing a group of people to oversee the well-being of its employees, the team takes on an air of importance, which conveys that the company takes health seriously. Employees can also see that they have senior-executive-sanctioned support in helping them achieve their wellness goals. Additionally, communicating the activities of the team will keep appointees engaged in the process and may maintain interest in the program.

The wellness team is only as strong as its leader. Without strong leadership, the group may lack direction, making achievement of program goals more difficult. What is important is that the leader engenders respect throughout the organization, has valuable management and communication skills, can set priorities and deadlines, and can motivate others effectively.

With strong leadership in place, it is also vitally important to have team members who represent all areas and levels of the organization. With a diverse group of people from many departments acting as team members, employees are likely to see the program as broad-based and egalitarian. In other words, they will see the company deliberately choosing people from throughout the organization to carry out the company's health mission, as opposed to selecting an elite few.

Having representative employees from all levels of the organization is also important to avoid what Hunnicutt calls an "'us versus them' impression whereby frontline employees think that wellness is only something reserved for the organization's elite." This means collaboration between frontline employees and senior executives is a must. Hunnicutt also underscores an important point: Not everyone on the team has to be in good health. In fact, by including people of differing health statuses, the company continues to underscore that the wellness program is inclusionary at all levels.

Two other important points to consider include scheduling regular wellness team meetings and the creation of a formal agenda. The team can start to meet monthly, and then as the program grows the meeting times can be moved to bi-monthly or even weekly. As the program matures, meetings can be conducted less frequently.

Meeting frequently establishes a rhythm and holds the interests of the team members. This rhythm establishes a cohesiveness and camaraderie that helps keep health priorities forward. Teams that work together and enjoy working collaboratively get things done much faster and more efficiently than those that meet only occasionally.

Formal agendas are one of the most effective ways to get and keep a meeting on track. They help focus the team on the items that need to be covered in the allotted time. Meetings without agendas tend to wander off-course and end with little accomplished.

Before the next meeting is conducted, all team members should be invited to contribute their ideas and tasks to the wellness leader for inclusion on the next meeting's agenda. By giving team members access to the agenda, and thereby giving voice to their input, more can be accomplished during and after the meetings. The agenda should be finalized and disseminated to all members well in advance of each meeting to allow for any needed preparation.

One task often overlooked is the keeping of minutes. According to Hunnicutt, thoughtful and detailed minutes can be extremely useful in recording and monitoring the team's activities and progress. It is often best to designate one person as "the minutes keeper" to maintain continuity. This is a position that could rotate every year.

Once the meeting is concluded, the minute keeper should prepare the minutes and distribute them to the group so that there is time to make corrections before the next meeting. As an added reminder, minutes might also be redistributed with the next agenda just to refresh people's memories.

Not only do detailed minutes keep track of the team's progress, but they also can be invaluable when new members join the team. The minutes will educate new members, as well as get them up to speed.

The team should also be encouraged to communicate frequently outside the regular wellness team meetings. These exchanges will aid in achieving goals, and build cooperation. However, formal communication should flow through channels that have already been created.

Lastly, Hunnicutt recommends that wellness team members consider ongoing continuing education as part of their role with the health management program. Continuing education opportunities are plentiful, in both classroom and online formats. Further, there are many opportunities for wellness team members to hear leading health experts speak on a wide variety of topics, through conferences, seminars, or more informal gatherings. Many of these venues are available through the Internet.

Also, disease management and wellness publications can be a rich source of information.

Health Library

With the plethora of health-related books, magazines, videos, and Internet-accessible information available today, you might consider installing a health and wellness library within your organization. A library can provide employees with the opportunity to access health and wellness

information at work, which can be viewed in the library or checked out to read on breaks.

A well-rounded library should include medical books for the layperson, books related to general and specific diseases and conditions, instructional audio tapes, DVDs, health magazines, and newsletters.

Publicize the library in all communication materials, and house the library in a high-traffic area. If it seems appropriate to your circumstances, install audio- and video-playing equipment so that employees can listen or watch right on the premises.

Best Coaching Practices

In-person coaching

Those employees who are considered low risk may self-direct to company health services. However, those employees who are at higher risk may need more intervention and support to help them make behavior changes. Although the program may offer classes and online support, in some cases a one-to-one relationship with a health counselor or wellness coach may work best.

Different from a personal trainer, who may focus on fitness and nutrition, a wellness coach works with the whole employee, assessing physical, mental, and emotional needs as they relate to health. A good health and wellness coach will take the time to ask questions, listen to concerns, and develop a personalized one-on-one relationship with employees. This partnership can make all the difference in helping employees register and stay active in the health management program, and as a result, health coaching has been a common component of the health management program.

Employees who may be reluctant to communicate with their doctor or friends about wanting to make a behavior change may talk to a wellness coach because of workplace encouragement. What's more, wellness coaches can support employees in either a work or a home environment in a holistic and collaborative manner. By taking the time to address diet, exercise, and other behaviors that impact wellness, employees are more likely to develop and stick to a plan, especially when accountability to the wellness coach for growth and change is expected.

Perhaps one of the greatest values of wellness coaching is the highly personal contact the coach provides, with plans and goals designed specifically for each person helping each meet his or her particular goals.

Health and wellness coaches also provide resources and recommendations that complement traditional medical care. These resources can include yoga, massage, and other body therapies, acupuncture, meditation, and a host of other healing modalities.

If lifestyle and behavior changes are needed, a wellness coach can support the employee in a gentle but firm and encouraging manner. Wellness coaches work independently, or with organizations that offer wellness services.

Telephone counseling

Some employees may not feel the need to have an in-person coach, but may still want the support of a caring person. In such cases, a telephone coach can be effective. By contracting with a reputable outside vendor that provides health coaches, you can provide the personal support some employees may need. There are other benefits of telephone-based health coaching. Employees who participate by telephone can arrange a convenient time and place to talk to the coach without the logistics of an in-person visit. Employees may also feel more comfortable and be more forthcoming on the phone because of the perceived anonymity.

Most telephonic coaching programs last six months to a year, though some last longer. Most have an intensive behavior change period, followed by a behavior maintenance component. By participating, employees can find themselves much further along in their behavior change efforts than they would have been on their own.

Of course, the primary objective of personal health coaching is to eliminate health risk factors.

With personal telephone coaching, it has been shown that approximately 45% to 50% of the risks can be improved or eliminated from the pool.

Given all of these benefits, telephone coaching for at-risk or high-risk employees is emerging as one of the more effective and preferred health management strategies. Telephone coaching should be considered an important component of the health management effort.

Employee assistance programs

A number of recent studies have demonstrated the value of including mental health efforts in a health management initiative, and employee assistance programs (EAPs) address these and other employee concerns. The development of the health management program provides an opportunity to integrate mental health activities with physical health activities, providing the program with a more comprehensive approach to address worker health.

For many individuals, mental health and physical health needs and issues tend to overlap. Integrating EAP and other mental health services with the physical health components of a health management effort can maximize the chances of success by treating the whole individual.

EAPs were first developed as a means to identify and support employees who were negatively affected by personal and professional problems.

Low- or no-cost services to employees can be offered in-house, usually through the human resources department, or they can be contracted through an outside vendor. The goal is to get troubled employees the help they need and get them back to doing productive work.

As EAPs have evolved they have begun to address more wellness-related concerns. The EAP may also become involved in disability-related issues as they relate to health. For example, workers recuperating from surgery or other injuries may become depressed at home. Financial issues may also plague the worker, causing stress.

If you have an EAP established, either in-house of contracted, it is wise to integrate it into the program. Someone from the EAP should sit on the wellness team and take part in the regular meetings.

By having the EAP more closely related to wellness services, some of the stigma associated with mental and behavioral health services will be diminished, and each program will be more successful than either could have been working separately.

These are just a few of the many online and in-person wellness tools that are available today. Separately, they can serve a useful purpose for a wide variety of employees who are challenged by differing health concerns. When included in the Health Import Model, they become building blocks of a comprehensive and integrated program that demonstrates a company's commitment to employee and dependent health. Employees will get the message and begin to experience the value of building support for good health into the company culture.

New tools for the future

Regardless of the program, its intent, or the message, there are new tools available. While some are in their infancy, they will reshape how health management is delivered.

Some of these tools include:

- **PDAs/Blackberrys.** Palm Pilots and similar devices will receive information designed to support behavior change and health improvement. Many people manage their lives from their PDAs, so managing their health using the device is practical.

- **The Web.** While there are many health applications on the Web today, it is likely the Web will support health in many new ways in the future. The Web will serve as an extensive network of information sharing and gathering, virtual support communities, and health records. The Web will make tailored messages available in ways we can only imagine today.

- **E-mail.** Whether it comes on a PDA or a computer, e-mail will continue to serve a

role in supporting good health and controlling disease. While Spam continues to be a concern, giving trusted sources the ability to provide information to end-users in a secure format will continue to play a role. Further, coaching and other interacting involving professional or peer support can easily be communicated by e-mail.

- **Automated voice.** Automated voice technology continues to improve and the programming has become more creative. It can be used to cost-effectively educate, remind, and encourage participants in a health management program.

- **Text messaging.** Text messaging shows great promise in health management. Nearly everyone carriers a cell phone, and thus most people can receive health support messages. Further, they can respond by typing in data or uploading through a Bluetooth device. For instance, diabetic patients can use Bluetooth-enabled glucometers to send their readings through their cell phone. An automated endocrinologist can access the reading and text back messages or request additional information. The feedback and direction of the participant is nearly immediate, reaching him or her during the teachable moment. Text messaging can be used in prevention in similar ways. For instance, weight and exercise can be logged, questions about food selections can be asked by the participant with nearly instantaneous answers provided back, and reminders on keeping behavior promises can be delivered directly to the participant (such as reminding about exercise time).

- **Remote monitoring.** Many technologies are being used to monitor people with chronic illnesses. Some of the same technologies are utilized in prevention. The technologies include phone, Web, Bluetooth, and many others. These technologies monitor vital information for persons with chronic illnesses, and dispatch help when needed. In prevention, there are now downloadable pedometers, GPS systems to monitor miles walked, calories burned during exercise, and a host of other products.

Chapter 5

Investing in Your Wellness Program

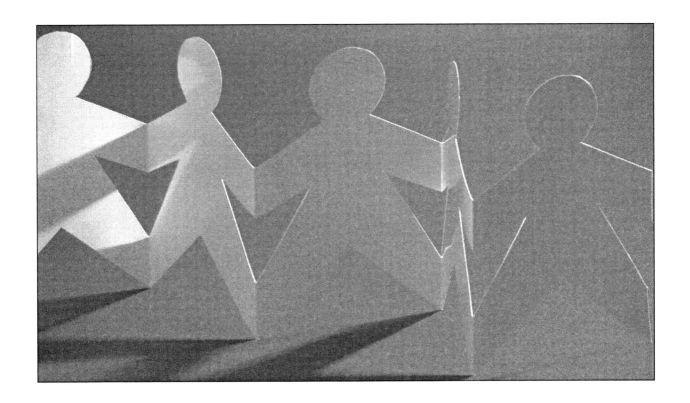

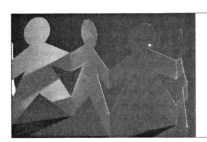

Investing in Your Wellness Program

An investment in people, in the form of a health management program, is an investment in your company's long-term health. In fact, a StayWell Communications study found that individuals who participated in health management programs were shown to reduce their use of disability benefits by as much as several days.

As we have illustrated in the preceding chapters, employees with chronic conditions and multiple health risks can cost a company thousands of dollars in additional healthcare costs. Many believe that the promotion of healthy lifestyles will ultimately save companies millions of dollars annually by getting at the root cause of chronic disease.

In the past, companies that have instituted health management programs have either underfunded them or not recognized them as a valuable business tool. This failure is usually a result of seeing a health management initiative as being outside the core of business, something almost superfluous to the more pressing needs of running the company.

In many cases, corporate America has been slow

to embrace health management programs in a meaningful way. The results of health management programs prove themselves over time. Further, they struggle with the basic question, "Can I change enough behaviors at a reasonable enough cost to generate a measurable ROI?"

In a recent survey by the Office of Disease Prevention and Health Promotion, only 17% of U.S. companies offering health promotion activities reported having a formally articulated set of goals and objectives. This lack of focused planning and lack of adequate investment dollars in health management programs can result in wasted time and cost.

For any department within an organization to function properly and produce positive results, some investment in staffing and resources is needed. A health management program is no exception. It does not require a significant amount of overhead. It does, however, require a reasonable budget, and without one it is unlikely your program will produce the results you and your employees seek.

Because health management programs are fairly new to most companies, especially small businesses, it can be hard to determine what an adequate budget is for a companywide health management effort. Depending on the size of the company and program, financial figures can vary widely from business to business, but as was stated earlier, they often range between $150 and $200 per employee per year.

Measuring ROI

Companies trying to determine the costs of creating a new department or initiative within the organization usually want to calculate the return on investment (ROI) of such a decision. However, because wellness programs are relatively new to the workplace and financial value on such programs is limited, determining ROI can be difficult. Accordingly, it is not surprising that the International Foundation of Employee Benefit Plans reported that 87% of employers surveyed that offer wellness programs acknowledged that they did not have concrete figures for ROI for their wellness initiatives. Fortunately, new strategies for estimating the ROI of health and wellness programs are emerging.

Recent research suggests that employers save, on average, $3 for every $1 spent on health initiatives. One study found that employers experienced a savings of $3.48 in reduced healthcare costs and $5.82 in lower absenteeism costs for every dollar

spent on employee wellness. Although these figures provide some range for an expected ROI, calculating an accurate ROI for a particular program depends on several variables, including the design of the program, the underlying health of the population, program participation, health behavior change, health outcomes improvement, employee turnover, the costs of incentives to encourage program participation and behavior change, and the cost of overhead. This chapter outlines some of the key considerations in developing an ROI as well as the most common methodology for calculating the health and wellness program's ROI.

Establishing a baseline

As a first step to determine the types of health and wellness programs that are needed companies frequently establish a baseline assessment of current and potential health-related costs. Health-related costs are not limited to medical costs, but also include disability claims, workers' compensation claims, and health-related productivity loss.

This integrated view allows an employer to answer the following questions:

- What are the company's most commonly occurring health problems?

- What are the most prevalent unhealthy behaviors and lifestyles that can lead to future health-related costs?

- What are the potential effects of these health problems on work performance, absence, industrial accidents, and disability?

- Where should the company target its health and wellness initiatives?

Considerations in calculating ROI

Early on, plan sponsors must determine whether to provide an incentive, and if so, what amount to provide, for program participation and outcomes improvement.

Generally, it is recommended that some funds be used to incent program participation and some to incentivize outcomes improvement. In either case, you should include in your total program cost the amount of the incentives to determine the ROI, and you should be careful up front not to establish so high an incentive that a positive ROI from the program becomes unlikely.

During program implementation, determine the data that will eventually be needed to determine the program's ROI. With proper planning, ROI is more easily measured and can be maximized.

A cost savings/cost avoidance component of a health management program ROI is health-related productivity. ROI opportunity exists when absenteeism and less than optimal presenteeism can be avoided. Health-related absenteeism is defined as not being physically present at work because of physical or mental health. Health-related presenteeism is defined as a reduction in an employer's performance when an employee comes to work when he or she is not physically or mentally performing at full capacity. Presenteeism usually takes the form of a reduction in the quality, quantity, or timeliness of work completed. It may also have financial safety, or other environmental consequences, depending on the type of job.

Wellness program costs

Buck Consultants, a leading human resources and benefits consulting firm, recently analyzed responses from 555 organizations representing almost 7 million employees. The resultant report, *WORKING WELL: A Global Survey of Health Promotion and Workplace Wellness Strategies*, found that respondents spent an average of $135 per employee per year on wellness programs, although some can spend as much as $500 per year. Respondents also reported spending an average of $100 per employee per year on incentive rewards, but that can exceed $500 per employee.

Interestingly, the Buck report also found that employers also indicated significant plans to expand their incentive programs in the next one to three years.

Presenteeism losses are typically measured via self-reporting. Absenteeism can often be measured through human resource records, although this is becoming more difficult since the advent of paid time off. During program design, it is important to determine how health-related productivity will be measured, including which validated instrument will be used to collect self-reported information, how frequently the data will be collected, and how measurement will be administered.

Calculating the ROI

Despite the challenges in measuring ROI for health and wellness, this measurement has become increasingly more important to justify the health management program.

At the most basic level, ROI is measured by the amount of savings generated divided by the cost of the program. The cost of the program will include the fees paid to the vendors for administering the program, the cost of any employee incentives provided, and any internal costs incurred by the employer. Savings can be calculated from actual medical and pharmacy claims data can be forecast based on changes in health risks as self-reported in an HRA. In either approach, the health-related productivity savings measured can be added to the total.

The forecasting approach is currently used more frequently because of the ability to more quickly estimate the ROI, the lower analytic cost of this approach relative to a claims analysis, and the difficulty in assessing which factors, besides the health and wellness program, contributed to the change in medical costs (e.g., benefit design changes). The typical methodology for the ROI forecasting model is to assess the change in risk over time for the participating group and, when possible, to compare the change to that of a non-participating control group.

Some of the more common health risks that are measured include the following:

- Body weight (body mass index or body fat percentage)

- Tobacco use

- Blood pressure

- Cholesterol

- Blood glucose level

- Excessive alcohol use

- Physical activity

- Stress reduction

Within that overall framework are several considerations for the ROI calculation. First, not every member starts the program in the same week or even the same month because of program ramp-up, new-member enrollment, and other factors. Thus, the length of time a participant has to participate in follow-up programming prior to completing a subsequent HRA will vary. Consequently, a cohort must be defined relative to the starting dates of the participants, typically two to three months following the close of the HRA participation window.

Once the group is determined (i.e., the study group), the risks can again be stratified following completion of the second HRA using the original risk thresholds to determine change at time two. The risks that were identified in the first HRA can stay the same, get worse, improve, or improve to the point of risk elimination. Two different approaches are commonly used in quantifying the risk change:

- Counts of risk elimination or development of a new risk based on a predetermined threshold (e.g., cholesterol < 200)

- Changes in risk levels (e.g., cholesterol improved 20 points from T1-T2)

In either case, risks that worsen/develop are counted against those that improve/are eliminated to determine not effect.

To determine a "normal" risk change for comparison, use eligible individuals who did not enroll in a coaching program as a control group if there are a sufficient number of them. If not, you can compare the T1-T2 trend to a similar employer

that is not offering a wellness initiative, but does not offer HRAs.

While neither of these constitutes a perfect control group, it is often the best approach possible outside a clinical setting.

Once you have determined changes in risk factors, you can assign a financial value to this change using one of several sources. Dr. Dee Edington, a researcher from the Health Management Research Center at the University of Michigan, and his colleagues have published a number of studies quantifying the value of cost of each risk factor. Likewise, the HERO study identified the costs associated with a number of key health risks. Ron Goetzel, a researcher at Brown University, has conducted other research and financial estimations.

When using estimated cost per risk, always adjust the dollar figures to the most recent year's dollars. Note that these values typically do not include health-related productivity savings, so any productivity value must be added.

In forecast studies, each individual is assigned a savings or loss based on his or her risk change and the specific costs associated with their respective risks. Program savings can be calculated by examining the differential savings between the T1 and T2 measures. If a comparison group is available, subtract the comparison group savings from the intervention group savings to arrive at a net savings. You can then divide the net savings by the program cost to estimate an ROI.

As mentioned earlier, when available, you can also include health-related productivity savings in the calculation. The methodology is similar to that for risk factor cost calculation. Calculate changes in productivity, both absenteeism and presenteeism, for each individual from T1 to T2, and assign a dollar value to that change. You may need to use an average salary for the entire work force, or ideally, you can use a salary specific to that individual. For any savings observed, subtract the productivity savings of the comparison group to arrive at net productivity savings, while addressing natural migration.

With the growing prevalence of unhealthy behaviors, the need for creative and effective health and wellness programs will continue to grow. As with any employer-funded benefit, it will be important to assess the ROI from such initiatives. Companies have multiple options for measuring the ROI; and with careful planning and analytic review as outlined in the preceding sections of this chapter, you can begin to determine the monetary value of these programs for your organization.

Program evaluation

Later, in Chapter 8, we will go into more depth about program evaluation; however, a few comments are warranted in this section because we are discussing how a wellness initiative might be considered an investment. Program evaluation is the process of reviewing the information available about the program and determining if health and cost outcome goals were met.

Earlier, we presented information on forecasting the approximate health-related impact of a program. With actual program evaluation, it is best to use actual longitudinal analysis. In such analyses, actual claims costs are reviewed rather than forecast.

When assessing the data, the National Wellness Institute (NWI) has identified three primary areas to consider:

- **Medical claims:** Collect the data that will allow you to compare your program's pre- and post-program costs for participants and nonparticipants.

- **Cost of sick leave:** NWI recommends taking the amount of sick leave used pre- and post-program and multiplying the difference by the cost of the average wage scale for that time period.

- **Cost of workers' compensation:** To determine this, NWI recommends dividing the total workers' compensation claims cost by the number of full-time employees that are covered by workers' compensation. This will give you a per-capita or per-employee workers' compensation cost. This will assist you in determining if the costs have changed after launching the health management program.

Knowing your costs and how they are changing over time will be valuable. However, they must be linked to the health management program to demonstrate the cause and effect impact. More of this will be discussed in Chapter 8.

The Role of Health Plans

Small businesses have been reluctant to spend the money on a wellness program because insurers have not responded with a direct premium reduction, but that may be changing. For example, Blue Shield of California offers Healthy Lifestyles Rewards, a program that rewards its customers' employees with cash and other prizes for filling out health questionnaires and engaging in healthy behavior.

The health insurer also went as far as to reward a California company for its health management program. Camico Mutual Insurance Company in Redwood, CA, offers wellness programs to its 100 employees. Because it collected data and saw results from the program, it asked its insurer, Blue Cross of California, for a break on health insurance premiums. Reluctant at first, Blue Cross agreed to allow Camico to offer a health savings account with more generous benefits to its employees. The health insurer also agreed to a

10% lower premium than it typically sells to a company of Camico's size.

Some of the nation's biggest health insurers, including WellPoint, United Health's PacifiCare, and Horizon Blue Cross, also offer wellness incentives. Insurance companies, although slow to regard wellness programs as part of their core scope of services, are now beginning to respond to increasing customer demand for these services. Additionally, these companies are recognizing that impacting behaviors can help them improve their eroding margins.

Recent research demonstrates why many health plans are taking health management more seriously. Studies show that employee absenteeism is reduced when wellness programs are implemented. In fact, a study at Prudential Insurance reported that disability days were 20% lower and disability-per-capita costs were 32% lower after implementing a wellness program. In addition, annual medical costs fell by 46%. According to a study of a wellness program at Providence General Medical Center, per-capita workers' compensation costs were reduced by 83%, with other savings realized in reduced sick leave and healthcare costs, thanks to the implementation of a wellness program.

These studies document tangible economic benefit from wellness programs, and insurance companies are starting to take notice and reward companies that are willing to initiate such programs.

Building a Wellness Budget

Having a sufficient budget to support your health management program is crucial to its success. Having a detailed and realistic budget is critical. Dr. Joseph A. Leutzinger, in his report, *Building Your Wellness Budget*, recommends three areas of budgeting that need focused attention: budget principles, budget justification, and budget sustainability. These constitute the foundation of a healthy and ongoing wellness program.

Budget principles

To be successful, each program component will have to be justified in terms of ROI, popularity, projected cost, and other important factors. Program expenses will decline over time, as some of the costs are first-year only. Thus, program participation costs are heaviest in the first two years.

Before developing a wellness budget, everyone involved with the program, from the person who oversees it to the highest-ranking executive, should be familiar with how the company will fund the health management initiative. Clarity on this in the beginning will eliminate much confusion and surprise later.

With this clarity, and with data collection to back up any decisions, one way to budget, according to Leutzinger, is to give the program a finite amount of money with which it must operate. Because many departments in companies all over the world must adhere to strict budget parameters, financially supporting a health management initiative in the same way will be familiar. The staff, educational materials, and technology should all be allotted a dollar value within the program and a budget determined from there.

Although this can be an effective way to begin to fund a wellness program, it is important to remember that expenses can grow over the years as the program becomes more popular, participation grows, and more programs are added. Typically, once this happens, finite budgets can shrink so that maintaining the program within set parameters can become more difficult over time. As with budgets in other departments, you will need to closely monitor the health management budget to keep pace with the program's needs.

Another way to approach wellness funding, according to Leutzinger, is the zero-based budgeting approach, with each program offering presented in an itemized budget. The upside is seeing that everything in the program has the chance of being adequately funded. The downside can be trying to pinpoint that number, without going over or under. An added bonus is the possibility of adding or eliminating components as a separate item. In other words, a component can be eliminated as a singular item, without affecting the whole budget.

Ideally, the way to fund your health management initiative is to have the program pay for itself.

One easy way to accomplish this is to charge an employee premium differential. For instance, employees not participating in the program pay a slightly higher health insurance premium than those in the program. Given the low cost of most programs the differential charge to nonpartici-pants more than covers the administrative/vendor program costs. Using this approach there is mini-mal risk given your ROI gain and other benefits of the program will actually start from the break-even point rather than having to recoup any sunk costs first.

Budget justification

Much of the discussion regarding budget justifica-tion will occur when discussing program ROI and what resources staff members need to produce the desired outcomes.

The steering committee should meet after the first year of operation and determine what constituted the health program's successes and near misses. Was it a success? What succeeded? What didn't do as well? Why? What has been the feedback of program components? What has been the feedback from the program overall? From this discussion, questions concerning budget renewal, justification of the previous year's budget, and justification of the overall program and its com-ponents will arise and be answered.

Budget justification after the first year will depend heavily on both the short-term results that have been monitored and the long-term success expect-ed from the program. Both are critical. Short-term results, such as flu vaccines, prenatal care, smoking cessation, weight loss programs, and productivity improvements, can appear within the first year. Long-term results, such as changes in the trend for chronic conditions, as well as getting employees to maintain a new healthy lifestyle, can be more difficult to determine in the short term.

But keeping track of short-term results, even for long-term programs, can provide justification for ongoing budget. *Budget sustainability equals program sustainability*: To sustain your wellness program, you will need to prove its worth every year through your evaluation process.

Taxes

They say there are only two absolutes in the world: death and taxes. Employers creating health man-agement programs will need to include tax issues in a budget plan, as well. This can be tricky, so a good tax attorney or accountant will be valuable in the process.

Tax issues can arise when employers pay for coverage that does not constitute "medical care." In addition, employers that link incentives or penalties to wellness initiatives can face a number of risks, ranging from legal claims to tax penalties for failing to properly report and withhold income and employment taxes.

Table 5.1 from the Department of Labor shows nontaxable and taxable benefits in most states as they relate to wellness programs. In addition to reviewing this table, it is prudent to check with a legal tax authority in your state to ensure tax compliance.

Table 5.1
Nontaxable and Taxable Benefits

Nontaxable Benefits	Taxable Benefits
The cost of an HRA	Cash incentives over a specific dollar amount
In-house use of a fitness facility	Large fitness equipment (treadmills or bicycles)
At-work health seminars or classes	Vitamins or supplements without a physician diagnosis and recommendation
Vouchers for the on-site cafeteria	Fitness memberships without a physician's diagnosis and recommendation
Smoking cessation or weight loss programs based on a physician's recommendation	

Source: Department of Labor.

The U.S. Department of Labor also stipulates that a wellness plan that fails to comply with the final regulations of the Health Insurance Portability and Accountability Act of 1996 can generally mean that the employer can be assessed excise taxes of up to $100 per day for each day the plan does not comply, for each participant in the plan to whom the failure relates. So, for example, a plan with 100 participants who are affected by the failure could expose an employer to a potential excise tax of $10,000 per day for each day of noncompliance. This tax may be excused for reasonable cause and is capped at 10% of the aggregate amount the employer paid for the group health plan during the preceding year, or $500,000, whichever is less. If, however, the noncompliance occurs before the IRS notifies the employer of its intent to audit the plan, and if the failure continues during the period being examined, the IRS will not excuse taxes below a certain minimum amount, even if the failure resulted from reasonable cause and was not due to willful neglect.

Faced with the risk of these excise taxes, companies that offer wellness programs should consult their tax attorneys or the Department of Labor when addressing their compliance issues to be aware of certain hidden pitfalls. The Department of Labor supplies a checklist that employers can go through to maintain compliance.

For example, one item requires the employer to determine whether the wellness program is part of a group health plan, which requires a determination of whether the program is subject to Part 7 of the Employee Retirement Income Security Act of 1974. The guidance offered in the checklist may not be sufficient for employers to correctly make this determination in every case. Another item requires the employer to determine whether the program, though discriminatory, is "saved by benign discrimination." This concept permits employers to design wellness plans that allow

discrimination in favor of an individual due to a health factor. Although examples are offered to shed light on the meaning of "benign discrimination," an employer is still required to apply this concept on a case-by-case basis to determine whether the program may avoid compliance with the wellness program standards.

In some states, a tax credit is extended to small-business employers that recognize the importance of worksite wellness. By bringing worksite wellness into the business, the employer has a unique opportunity to provide a healthy workplace for its employees, while utilizing this tax credit. Again, check current state tax laws to determine whether a program qualifies.

By considering the aforementioned points as you design and implement your health management program, you can ensure that the program will operate efficiently while avoiding operational and financial pitfalls. Using a holistic approach in the measurement, data collection, evaluation, health insurance, budgeting principles, and tax planning, you can assure that your health management program gets off on the right foot and grows with your company.

Chapter 6

Implementing an Effective
Health Management Program

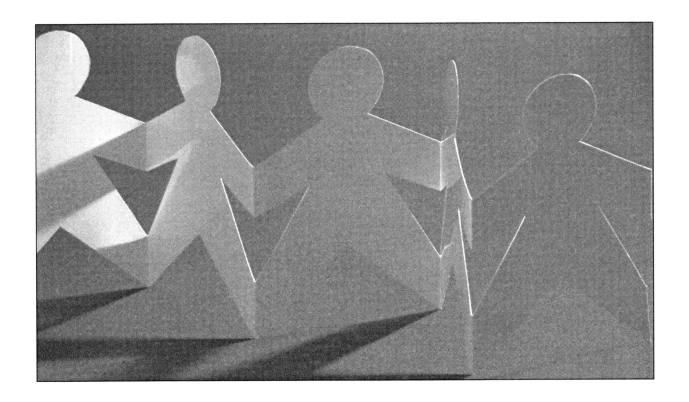

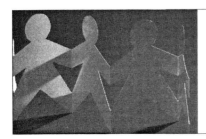

Implementing an Effective Health Management Program

As we mentioned in Chapter 2, before implementing your health management program, senior management must be on board. This will ultimately result in your company culture supporting healthy behavior. You must also establish an effective communications plan. Finally, you must develop an implementation plan that outlines the key steps that must be completed to successfully launch and operate. This plan also should outline the dates by which steps must occur to keep the program coordinated and on track.

Doing these things will maximize the chances your program will be launched effectively and that the program will be successful over time.

Senior Management Support

Without strong senior management support, it is doubtful a health management initiative will survive, let alone thrive. This support must start from the top with the CEO and other senior management. These executives play a critical role in communicating the value of health management throughout the organization. Senior management support helps to ensure that the rest of the work force will fully embrace the initiative and will dedicate the resources to make it successful.

CEO support

One of the most important factors in building and maintaining an effective health management program is having executive management buy-in, particularly the support of the CEO and other senior management.

Employees in the organization take many of their behavioral cues from their supervisors, managers, and executive leaders. If the leadership does not fully support the health management initiative, chances are the employees won't either. Employees know when executive management is being genuine and when they are just going through the motions. Those CEOs and executives who wholeheartedly embrace the value of health management will have a much easier time sparking employee interest. Openly being a role model for healthy habits is even more impressive.

During program development, CEOs can benefit from talking to other CEOs who have already established similar programs within their companies. This peer-to-peer discussion helps to avoid pitfalls, and provides reassurance that a health management initiative is being used as a successful business tool. It is also an opportunity to establish a benchmarking partner.

In addition, other resources are available. The Washington, DC-based policy group Partnership for Prevention and the U.S. Chamber of Commerce have published *Leading by Example* (*www.prevent.org*), which highlights testimonials from CEOs of large, medium, and small companies that have launched health management programs. Their support and feedback can prove to be valuable in initial as well as ongoing stages of program development.

If senior leadership needs more information before deciding to launch a health management program, numerous studies have been published and case studies written that provide objective information. Journals in which this information is most likely to be found include: *The Journal of Occupational and Environmental Medicine*, the *American Journal of Health Promotion*, and the publications of the American College of Sports Medicine and the Institute for Health and Productivity Management. You can find other case studies on the Internet by searching on *Google.com* or *Yahoo.com*.

If firsthand experience is beneficial in gaining the support of senior management, enrollment in an executive health program may be an option. Many well-known hospitals and medical centers offer such programs to executives. Usually requiring no more than one day to complete, these personal, hands-on programs designed specifically for executives emphasize the importance and value of maintaining good health. Relatively painless, these comprehensive health programs offer full physicals and educational support. Many CEOs of companies with leading health management initiatives have cited participation in an executive health program as part of what influenced their decision to launch a companywide effort.

Supervisor accountability

Until managers are held at least partially accountable for health programming in their departments, few employees will take up the mission with full seriousness or commitment. In environments where managers have been held accountable for safety, significant improvements have been made. Similar accountability is required for the support and delivery of a health management effort.

Supervisors should be trained to understand and effectively support the health management program, similar to how employee assistance programs train supervisors to recognize family challenges, substance abuse, or other personal problems that could affect the worker and the work environment. In some cases, wellness retreats have even been used to give supervisors firsthand experience. Supervisors can be taught to recognize emerging health problems and to provide assistance and referral, as needed. Given the privacy laws of the Health Insurance Portability and Accountability Act of 1996 and similar legislation, managers must learn to exercise caution in how they approach their role.

To help supervisors fully grasp, accept, and carry out the health management initiative, managers should learn their responsibilities in supporting the health management program. These responsibilities might include:

- Delivering program information to employees

- Facilitating basic health culture improvements

- Encouraging employees to participate in the health risk assessment (HRA) and other wellness initiatives

- Outwardly supporting the health management initiative

In many cases, supervisors are in the best position to see when health issues are affecting performance and to take direct or indirect action to address those issues using tools provided by the health management program. By being part of the frontline defense system, supervisors can aid in identifying and helping to resolve many health

problems before they became irreversible. This support will help the employee stay healthy, improve work performance, and potentially reduce cost.

To hold supervisors accountable in a more formal way, a percentage of each manager's performance appraisal can be based on his or her success in carrying out health management responsibilities. This sets a tone within the culture that health management is an important component of business success.

It is imperative that executive management participate and continue to support the health management program. As we have stated, employees often take their cues from the behavior of management. If executives are participating in HRAs and other wellness programs, employees will follow their lead.

Establishing a Wellness Culture

A supportive environment is critical to your health management program's launch and ongoing success. A company culture is established over many years. To change it, even in small ways, takes time and involves making health a part of the company's mission. Also required are senior executive support, teamwork, consistent and constant communication, company policy changes, and the monitoring of progress.

A cultural framework

A white paper produced by Health Enhancement Systems and written by Dr. Judd Allen, president, Human Resources Institute, provides a good primer on the subject of culture and how it can support wellness. In this white paper, Allen presents "Normative Systems" as a common construct for understanding culture. This topic is explored more completely in Allen's book, *The Organizational Unconscious: How to Create the Corporate Culture You Want and Need*, Second Edition. This cultural construct includes five elements: shared values and priorities, norms, touch points, peer support, and work climate. Together these factors drive behavior choices.

Shared values and priorities

Most corporate cultures value things, such as profitability, customer service, and innovation. In a company with a healthy culture, well-being is also included, emphasizing that healthy people are essential to the overall business strategy. Clearly identifying employee health as an organizational value makes a strong statement.

Norms

Norms are social expectations for behavior and beliefs. More simply put, they are "the way we do things around here." A wellness culture makes it easier for people to live healthy lifestyles by supporting physical activity during breaks, healthy food options in the cafeteria, and stress management breaks throughout the day. Although such a culture does not ridicule people who do not follow healthy lifestyle practices, it does make it harder and less acceptable. Changing the norms takes time, often two to four years, but it can be done. Some changes can take hold almost immediately. You can measure improvement in norms over time using cultural audits, such as those provided by the Human Resources Institute.

Touch points

Touch points are used to establish and maintain norms. They occur by formal policy, procedures, and programs, as well as through informal means. Allen points out that those policies that promote work-life balance can occasionally be offset when burning the midnight oil is required by providing praise for going the extra mile. Touch points might include the following:

- **Modeling:** people and actions serving as role models, as well as visible removal of old models that were previously acceptable but have no place in the new culture

- **Rewards and recognition:** rewarding healthy behavior while taking care not to mistakenly reward unhealthy behavior

- **Confrontation:** appropriate reaction from people when they observe healthy versus unhealthy behavior

- **Recruitment and selection:** the evidence of, and emphasis on, healthy behavior during the hiring process

- **Orientation:** the evidence of and emphasis on healthy behavior in the early stages of employment

- **Training:** reinforcing healthy behavior as people learn in the organization

- **Rites, symbols, and rituals:** regular events that remind and support people in living healthy behaviors and avoidance of events that are destructive

- **Communication:** information, feedback, and attention focused on healthy behavior

- **Relationship development:** relationships that form around healthy behavior practices rather than unhealthy ones (e.g., a walking club versus a pub night)

- **Resource commitment:** use of time, money, and other resources to demonstrate commitment to healthy behaviors

To establish proper touch points, build on existing strengths. Begin by addressing enough touch points to tip the balance, and involve employees in the decision-making.

Peer support

Peer support involves assistance from friends, family, coworkers, and supervisors in living a healthy lifestyle. Also valuable are the formal health management programs that were discussed throughout this book.

Work climate

In an article published by Allen in a 1987 issue of the *American Journal of Health Promotion*, he identifies three cultural climate factors that play a central role in the intersection of organizational development and personal wellness. When these factors do not exist, employees may be so distracted by distrust, anger, and negativity that they are unable to focus on their own healthy behaviors. These climate factors include:

- **Sense of community:** a feeling of belonging, trust, caring, and mutual understanding

- **Shared vision:** a shared understanding, role, and stake in the achievement of success

- **Positive outlook:** a workplace that thrives with optimism and enthusiasm

Wellness programs can play a central role in work climate by establishing a sense of community around healthy practices, supporting new organizational initiatives and challenges, and investing in people who remain optimistic and embrace self-improvement.

Improving the culture

Allen outlines four primary steps that must be taken to actively change the culture to one that supports healthy behaviors. These steps are:

1. **Preparation:** Analyze the current culture, set objectives, and develop leaders throughout the organization.

2. **Involvement:** Introduce the vision of the new culture to all levels of the organization, giving them ample opportunity to embrace it and use it as a springboard for personal development.

3. **Integration:** Align the culture and create touch points by announcing new policies, procedures, and the implementation of new programs.

4. **Sustainability:** Evaluate progress, celebrate success, renew efforts that need attention, and extend the culture further.

Employees at all levels have a role in changing culture. Although senior leadership support is essential, employees throughout the organization see the existing subcultures, can help to keep the plan for cultural change organized, are useful in avoiding pitfalls, and can be enthusiastic role models at the grassroots level. To formalize the involvement of all levels of employees, often wellness teams are utilized.

Program Communications

Effectively communicating the health management program to all employees is vital to the program's success. The health management effort must be recognized by all employees, and they must understand its importance, its value, and

what it has to offer. One of the best ways to do this is by branding the program with an identity and a message that are an integral part of the company's mission. By identifying and communicating the program as a unique yet serious and vital component of the overall business strategy, you will ensure that employees will eventually come to treat wellness as part of their work life.

For greatest success, you must implement a comprehensive marketing and promotion plan and aim it at all levels of the organization. Similar to any good advertising initiative, the plan should recognize and target the different constituencies within the company. For instance, some portions of the communications plan should be focused on senior-level management while other portions should be focused on supervisors who must be supportive in allowing employees to take time to participate in on-site events (when appropriate). Other parts of the plan should focus on individual workers and dependents to encourage their participation in programming. Buy-in and enthusiasm from all of these subgroups will be necessary for the program to be successful.

Health management programming must be effectively sold to employees and their dependents. With an effective communications plan in place, you will maximize the chances that your employees will hear the message, understand it, and, most important, act on it.

Constant message

To create a culture in which good health is valued by everyone in the organization, the company must make the health management program a constantly visible part of every employee's workday. This will require that you develop a consistent message for the overall initiative as well as for every component of the program. Constantly delivering the message through a variety of media will reinforce the importance of taking action and being vigilant in maintaining good health. Employees and dependents seeing the health management program message must become the rule, not the exception. To achieve this, consider the following.

Kickoff address

A kickoff address by the CEO is one of the most important preliminary communications vehicles for the program. Having the CEO launch the initiative through a companywide address gives the health management program tremendous support and credibility.

In the address, the CEO has the opportunity to personally reveal all the components of the health management program, including its guiding mission and values, the guidelines that will need to be followed for screenings and incentives, and the expectation that everyone will participate—including senior management.

This address will also provide the opportunity for all employees to have their questions and concerns addressed, by either the CEO or other senior managers, in a supportive environment. The address will highlight the broad-based support within the organization, including the inclusion of employee health as a value in the corporate mission. The open communication by the CEO will help the health management program and all its components to be viewed as part of the mainstream business effort.

Program kickoff

Plan a "kickoff" campaign to explain and generate interest in the health management initiative. This campaign should focus on the new program, its philosophy, mission, and goals, desired results, and benefits for every part of the organization. In particular, this kickoff campaign should answer the question for employees and dependents, "What is in it for me?"

The kickoff campaign should:

- Focus on tying together all program components

- Demonstrate the value of involvement

- Reinforce the fact that employees and dependents may begin participating in the program at any time

- Explain details of the HRA, other screenings, and how they may be taken

- Explain how to access Web and other electronic media

- Explain the programs and activities offered and how to enroll in them

- Outline the incentive program

- Reinforce confidentiality

The kickoff campaign is a good time to implement the use of various communications vehicles in announcing the program, through which you will continue to advertise its offerings.

Sending a letter to the homes of all employees announcing the program and providing all necessary information is a method of communication that has proven valuable in program kickoffs. In this way, dependents that might otherwise not be aware of the program have a better chance of seeing the information, supporting their spouse's participation, and getting involved personally.

The media used in the campaign should include:

- Brochures

- Banners in the facilities

- Posters

- Voice mail and e-mail from senior management to target groups

- A kickoff address to employees by the CEO (discussed earlier)

- Any other appropriate avenues for communication within your organization

Ongoing use of existing communications vehicles

Most organizations have a number of existing avenues for communication that can be utilized for promoting a health management program. Employee newsletters, benefits communications, safety communiqués, and broadcast e-mails or voice mails are all examples. A well-planned effort to continually utilize these resources can result in effective and cost-efficient communication.

Direct-to-consumer promotion

Keep in mind that health management programs, like any product, must use advertising to reach its intended audience in a way, and at a time that generate the intended action. As your health management program matures, more will be known about employee likes and dislikes, as well as the effectiveness of various forms of promotion in engaging potential participants, keeping them involved, and motivating them to achieve outcomes. As this occurs, you can make adjustments to your approach.

You can use certain program elements to focus on your targets. The HRA, for instance, will identify persons with specific needs so that at the right time, targeted information can be directed to them in an effort to mobilize them into action.

Providing personal success stories, or testimonials with the participant's identity protected (unless permission is provided), can provide powerful messages that will motivate workers to participate and achieve desirable health outcomes.

As in any form of direct-to-consumer advertising, touching the individual in a way that is most applicable to her or him often has the greatest effect.

Program posters and fliers (electronic and paper)

You can develop posters and fliers that promote the overall health management initiative as well as upcoming events. You can place these in locations to reach the proper audience. Although there are many ways to present information electronically, old-fashioned paper can also be effective, even though it is more expensive. Posters and fliers can communicate messages such as:

- Fitness and nutritional facts

- Information on upcoming or ongoing programs

- Information on notable national health days, such as World Health Day or The Great American Smokeout

- Recognition of individual employee achievements, or incentives earned (with the permission of the participant)

- Aggregate results of the program to date

All materials should include a program name and logo, both of which could be selected through a companywide contest to help gain employee buy-in. Physical locations for placing posters should include main entrance interiors, cafeterias, near time clocks, restrooms, and other high-traffic areas, or other places where workers gather. Electronic locations could be on the company home page, on the intranet site, or even be part of the e-mail template.

The use of marketing collateral

When communicating the health management initiative and all of its components, keep it light and interesting! The use of balloons, stickers, flowers, and music creates an enjoyable atmosphere for health fairs, screening activities, or education programs. Although health management is serious business, too sterile an approach can make participation intimidating.

Promotion through technology

One of the most cost-efficient ways to promote the wellness program is through online portals, voice mail, and e-mail. You should develop health program messages specifically for these vehicles and launch them accordingly. Sending an e-mail blast to every employee about an upcoming class or program ensures that everyone has exposure to the message. An occasional companywide voice mail can also be effective. To avoid having electronic messages be perceived as spam, you should use these tools judiciously.

Utilizing the company's intranet page for consistent information and news about employee health and the program can be one of the most effective ways to keep employees informed. Furthermore, providing health information on the intranet increases the credibility of the message and positions participation in the health management program as a normal part of doing business in the organization.

Annual report

Many of the aforementioned suggestions are aimed at internal employee communication. However, once your program is a success, sharing the results with outside parties demonstrates your commitment to health and the value you place on it as a vibrant entity. One of the best ways to communicate your results is through the company's annual report. This will help to feature the overall program to outsiders, to spotlight its achievements, and to help employees continue to understand the importance of health and wellness. Most annual reports address progress on major company objectives, and if your organization has made a full commitment, health management will fall under one or more of the objectives. The health

management program, like any other area of the business operation, will be measured by objective and key indicators tracked regularly by management. You can present progress on these key indicators as part of the annual report.

Utilizing an outside firm

If the internal capability or capacity to effectively design and implement a communications plan for your health management program does not exist, one option is to hire an outside firm to develop the plan and create and disseminate the components. Various vendors specialize in the delivery of these services.

Public relations firms, advertising specialty companies, and some health programming consulting groups will be able to provide the kinds of materials and guidance you will need to help you market a successful program. And because they have often already developed similar materials for other clients, these vendors can serve you cost-efficiently while still providing customized communications.

As a result, you may find that "outsourcing" your communications component is the most effective and cost-efficient approach.

Plan of Implementation

Most health management programs are developed over the course of six to 12 months and then are launched over an additional six to 12 months. Many tasks and activities must be coordinated for a program to be launched and operated effectively.

Program operations

It is common for organizations to appoint an executive steering committee to oversee the operations of the health management program. This group meets regularly to set the program's direction, and to make certain it stays on course. Usually, executives from across the enterprise are included on this team.

In addition to a steering committee, one or more employees are required to operate the program on a day-to-day basis. Where this staff reports within the organization varies among companies, but it is common to report to compensation and benefits, human resources department, the office of the medical director, or health and safety. The role of this employee or team is to effectively and efficiently operate the health management program in a way that gets all levels of management and employees fully engaged. The head of this staff should be the health management coordinator, who is accountable for meeting the program's objectives.

By providing a designated staff, the program will receive the attention it needs to be effective. Additionally, staff members will be viewed as a nucleus of support throughout the organization that other employees can go to with fresh opinions and ideas. A grassroots team of lay leaders can also provide assistance as was discussed in Chapter 2

Plan of implementation

To most effectively plan and operate a health management program you should establish an implementation plan. Often, this plan is documented in spreadsheet software such as Microsoft Excel, or in special project management software such as Microsoft Project. Major task groups as well as step-by-step subtasks are identified, and dates are specified by which each task must be completed. More sophisticated software even allows tasks that have interdependencies to be linked.

Some of the major task areas often documented include:

- Strategic planning

- Communications

- Data management

- Health assessment

- Web programming

- Fitness center networks

- Health coaching

- Disease management

- Incentive programming

- Measurement and evaluation

- Reporting

Establishing a series of subtasks in each of these areas and completing each systematically will result in the health management program being delivered on time and with high quality.

So, take the time necessary to get senior management on board. Prime your culture to support healthy behavior, and establish a plan to communicate the initiative effectively. Then, carefully plan the health management program and document the course you will take.

By doing so, you will ensure that initial acceptance of the program will be higher, participation will meet or exceed your objectives, ongoing enthusiasm for health management will be maintained, and the program will achieve better outcomes.

Chapter 7

Legal Issues

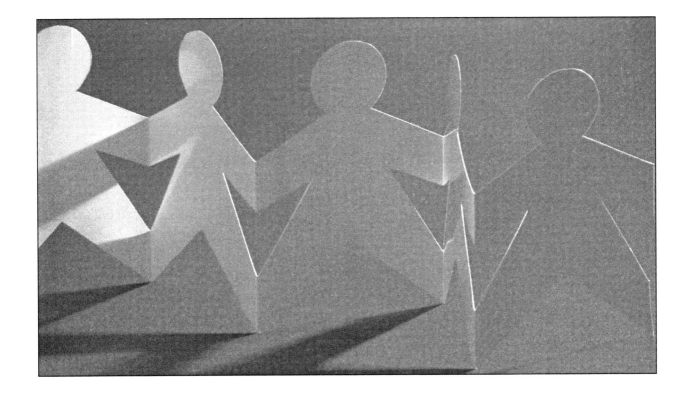

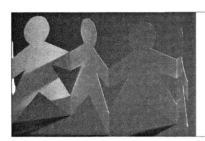

Legal Issues

When implementing a companywide health management program, you must consider legal issues that may impact your organization and employees. You must understand the Health Insurance Portability and Accountability Act of 1996 (HIPAA), the Americans with Disabilities Act of 1990 (ADA), and various federal and state laws as you plan and launch your health management program. Familiarity with these laws and other pending legislation is prudent. In addition, legal compliance issues may arise under:

- The Age Discrimination in Employment Act (ADEA)

- The Consolidated Omnibus Budget Reconciliation Act of 1985 (COBRA)

- The Employee Retirement Income Security Act of 1974 (ERISA)

- Various tax laws

HIPAA

HIPAA has detailed provisions that relate to company health management programs. These provisions spell out what companies can and cannot do when implementing and maintaining wellness programs, especially as it pertains to the use of personal health information and incentives.

In general, HIPAA requires that protected health information (PHI) for any individual participant be kept confidential, and sets a number of other legal rules concerning confidentiality and the use and handling of confidential information. This portion of the law is complicated by the fact that various entities delivering elements of the health management program and, therefore, handling PHI, may be defined as a healthcare provider whereas others may not. Healthcare providers have special and, often, more stringent requirements. Also, anyone receiving data could function as a business associate, requiring that he or she protects PHI in specified ways. Although the intent of HIPAA is to protect the public, it does provide challenges in the delivery of health management initiatives.

In 2006, the U.S. Department of Labor, the U.S. Department of Health and Human Services, and the U.S. Department of Treasury issued final regulations that addressed the nondiscriminatory provisions of HIPAA as they pertain to wellness programs. These regulations became effective February 12, 2007, and they apply to company benefit plan years beginning on or after July 1, 2007. Calendar-year benefit plans had to begin applying the regulations by January 1, 2008.

At its core, the HIPAA nondiscrimination provisions generally prohibit group health plans (including self-insured companies) from charging similarly situated individuals different premiums or contributions, or imposing different deductible, copayment, or other cost-sharing requirements, based on health factors. These factors include health status, medical condition (including both physical and mental illnesses), claims experience, receipt of healthcare, medical history, genetic information, and evidence of insurability, including conditions arising out of acts of domestic violence and disability.

In addition, the Department of Labor has ruled that any wellness program that provides a reward or penalty based on the ability to meet a health standard must meet five requirements to comply with nondiscrimination rules:

- Limit the reward or penalty to 20% of the value of the healthcare benefit.

- Be reasonably designed to promote health or prevent disease.

- Give eligible individuals the opportunity to qualify for the reward at least once per year.

- Show an annual qualification requirement.

- Be available to all similarly situated participants. For example, individually tailored program adjustments may be required for individuals who cannot meet health standards.

In addition, a notice that individual accommodations can be made for persons who could not otherwise meet the requirement due to a medical condition or for whom the requirement could be medically inadvisable must be provided.

The five requirements

Limit the reward or penalty to 20% of the cost of plan coverage, which is determined based on the total amount of employer and employee contributions.

For example, let's say the annual premium for employee-only coverage is $3,600; for family coverage, the premium is $9,000. If the wellness program is available to employees only, the reward cannot exceed $720 ($3,600 x 20%). If the program is available to any class of dependents, the reward cannot exceed $1,800 ($9,000 x 20%).

Rewards can be in the form of a discount or rebate of a premium or contribution, a waiver of all or part of a cost-sharing mechanism (e.g., deductibles, copayments, coinsurance), the absence of a surcharge, or the value of a benefit that would otherwise not be provided under the plan.

The program is reasonably designed to promote health and prevent disease.

Although a scientific record that a method promotes wellness is not needed, the wellness program must have a reasonable chance of improving the health of, or preventing disease in, participants and "must not be overly burdensome." Additionally, the program must not be a subterfuge for discriminating, based on a health factor, and must not be highly suspect in the method chosen to promote health or prevent disease.

The program gives individuals eligible to participate the opportunity to qualify for the reward at least once per year.

This requirement is fairly straightforward and points to the necessity of having good record-keeping from the start of program implementation. The rule is designed to provide participants regular opportunities to requality for a benefit based on self-improvement.

The reward is available to all similarly situated individuals.

The program must allow a reasonable alternative standard, or a waiver of the initial standard, for obtaining the reward to anyone who may find the initial program unreasonably difficult because of a medical condition. This also applies if obtaining the initial reward would be deemed medically

inadvisable. It is important to note that a specific alternative standard does not have to be established beforehand. It is sufficient to determine one once a participant informs you of the need.

For example, let's say employees who achieve a count of less than 200 on their yearly cholesterol test receive a 20% discount. An employee for whom it is medically difficult to achieve that number may be allowed to follow his or her doctor's advice of taking prescription medication and having periodic blood tests as a reasonable alternative. By following this plan, the employee would still be able to qualify for the discount.

It is legal, however, to seek verification (e.g., a doctor's statement) that a health factor makes it unreasonably difficult or medically inadvisable for an employee to achieve the initial standard.

Plan materials describing the terms of the program must disclose the availability of a reasonable alternative standard, or the possibility of a waiver of the initial standard.

This disclosure is not required in wellness plan materials that merely mention that a program is available, without describing its terms. To be safe, however, it is advisable to use language emphasizing the availability of reasonable standards, such as "If it is unreasonably difficult due to a medical condition for you to achieve the standards for the reward under this program, or if it is medically inadvisable for you to attempt to achieve the standards for this reward, call us at [phone number] and we will work with you to develop another way to qualify for the reward." Once you have settled on program language, check with your legal department to make sure it meets regulations.

Although many HIPAA regulations are exacting, there are some *exceptions* to HIPAA rules regarding wellness incentive plans, as well. Wellness programs do not have to comply with HIPAA provisions if:

- Participation in the program is made available to all similarly situated individuals

- None of the conditions for obtaining a reward under a wellness program is based on an individual satisfying a standard related to a health factor

- No reward is offered

Some examples of these exceptions might include:

- A program that reimburses all or part of the cost for memberships in a fitness center

- A diagnostic testing program that provides a reward for participation rather than for outcomes

- A program that encourages preventive care by waiving the copayment or deductible requirement for the costs of, for example, prenatal care or well-baby visits

- A program that reimburses employees for the costs of smoking cessation programs without regard to whether the employee quits smoking

- A program that provides a reward to employees for attending a monthly health education seminar

Keep in mind that other legal implications also pertain to the offering of rewards and incentives. These encompass such things as:

- Employees participating in testing, regardless of outcome

- Waiver of copayments and deductibles for prenatal programs

- Reimbursement of health club memberships

- Reimbursement for smoking cessation or weight management programs, regardless of outcome

- Filling out health risk and other screening assessments

Incentives are often an exceptional motivator for employees to enroll and participate in a health management program. Just make sure they meet federal and state guidelines.

Know your company's health plan

It's important to remember that under HIPAA, an employee cannot be denied eligibility for benefits or charged more for coverage because of any health factor, according to the U.S. Department of Labor. These health factors include health status, physical and mental medical conditions, claims experience, receipt of healthcare, medical history, genetic information, evidence of insurability, and disability.

Knowing what your health plans provide each employee and how they impact health management initiatives is a key to staying compliant. Health plans differ, so confirmation from your human resources and legal departments before launching health management efforts will help to ensure that the program is doing all it can, while staying within legal guidelines. Some things to keep in mind, according to the U.S. Department of Labor, include the following:

- A group health plan may not require an individual to pass a physical exam for enrollment, even if the individual is a late enrollee.

- A plan can require an individual to complete a healthcare questionnaire to enroll, provided that the health information is not used to deny, restrict, or delay eligibility or benefits, or to determine individual premiums.

- Group health plans may exclude coverage for a specific disease, limit or exclude benefits for certain types of treatments or drugs, or limit or exclude benefits based on a determination that the benefits are

experimental or medically unnecessary. But this applies only if the benefit restriction pertains uniformly to all similarly situated individuals and is not directed at individual participants or beneficiaries based on a health factor they may have. Plan amendments that apply to all individuals in a group of similarly situated individuals, and are effective no earlier than the first day of the next plan year after the amendment is adopted, are not considered to be directed at individual participants and beneficiaries.

- A plan cannot charge individuals with histories of high claims more than similarly situated individuals, based on their claims experience. In fact, group health plans cannot charge an individual more for coverage than other similarly situated individuals based on any health factor. Distinctions among groups of similarly situated participants in a health plan must be based on bona fide employment-based classifications consistent with the employer's usual business practice. Distinctions cannot be based on any of the health factors noted earlier, other than under the circumstances for wellness programs presented earlier. For example, part-time and full-time staff members, employees working in different geographic locations, and employees with different dates of hire or lengths of service can be treated as distinct groups of similarly situated individuals, with different eligibility provisions, different benefit restrictions, or different costs, provided that the distinction is consistent with the employer's usual business practice.

- In addition, a plan generally may treat participants and beneficiaries as two separate groups of similarly situated participants. The plan also may distinguish between beneficiaries based on, for example, their relationship to the plan participant, such as spouse or dependent child, or on the age or student status of dependent children. In any case, a plan cannot create or modify a classification directed at individual participants or beneficiaries, based on one or more of the health factors.

The HIPAA nondiscrimination provisions generally prohibit group health plans from charging similarly situated individuals different premiums or contributions or imposing different deductible, copayment, or other cost-sharing requirements based on a health factor.

However, as discussed earlier, there is the exception that allows plans to offer wellness programs. If none of the conditions for obtaining a reward under a wellness program is based on an individual satisfying a standard related to a health factor, or if no reward is offered, the program complies with the nondiscrimination requirements, assuming that participation in the program is made available to all similarly situated individuals.

For a group program that offers a reward to individuals who participate in voluntary testing for early detection of health problems, the plan does not have the right to use the test results to determine whether an individual receives a reward or the amount of an individual's reward. The plan's program does not base any reward on the outcome of the testing. Thus, it is allowed under the HIPAA nondiscrimination provisions, without being subject to the five requirements for wellness programs that do require satisfaction of a standard related to a health factor.

This also applies to plans offering a reward based on an individual's ability to stop smoking. Medical evidence suggests that smoking may be related to a health factor. The Diagnostic and Statistical Manual of Mental Disorders, which states that nicotine addiction is a medical condition, supports that position. In addition, a report of the U.S. Surgeon General adds that scientists in the field of drug addiction agree that nicotine, a substance common to all forms of tobacco, is a powerfully addictive drug.

For a group health plan to maintain a premium differential between smokers and nonsmokers, and not be considered discriminatory, the plan's nonsmoking program would need to meet the five directives that require satisfaction of a standard related to a health factor.

The program must accommodate individuals for whom it is unreasonably difficult to quit using tobacco products because of addiction by providing a reasonable alternative standard. This can include a discount in return for attending educational classes or for trying a nicotine patch. Plan materials describing the terms of the premium differential must make employees and dependents aware of the availability of a reasonable alternative standard to qualify for the lower premium.

As you can see, HIPAA guidelines for wellness programs can be somewhat complicated, and it is highly recommended that you seek expert counsel before launching your companywide health management initiative.

The ADA

The ADA does not specifically address health management programs in its guidelines. However, the ADA does weigh in when it comes to health issues and medical exams. Also remember that a company's self-insured health plan is considered a group health plan.

According to the Department of Health and Human Services, nothing in the ADA prohibits employers or health insurers from implementing health management programs that are focused on promoting good health and disease prevention. The ADA does prohibit denying qualified individuals, on the basis of disability, an equal opportunity to participate in or receive benefits under programs or activities conducted by employers.

Whether a wellness program that offers employee rewards or discounts for weight loss or for maintaining a certain body mass index violates the ADA will depend on how the program is designed and implemented. Under the proposed HIPAA nondiscrimination regulations, employers are permitted to offer discounts or rebates in return for employees' adherence to health promotion and disease prevention.

The HIPAA regulations for wellness programs describe a wide range of things that comply with the HIPAA nondiscrimination requirements, without having to satisfy any additional standards, including ADA. In addition, employers have flexibility in designing wellness programs that require employees to meet certain biometric risk factor thresholds or observe specific behaviors. They are offered this flexibility in return for rewards that could include discounts to personal health plan premiums under HIPAA's nondiscrimination requirements, if certain requirements are met.

One of the requirements is the reasonable alternative standard. As discussed earlier, the reasonable alternative standard requires employers to make an alternative standard available to individuals for whom it is unreasonably difficult to meet the initial standard, or for whom it is medically inadvisable to do so. The ADA refers to these types of accommodations as *reasonable accommodations*.

Under the proposed HIPAA regulations for wellness programs, employers and health plans have considerable flexibility in designing health management initiatives. That flexibility is useful in designing wellness programs that are permissible under the ADA.

However, employers and health plans should be aware that compliance with the proposed HIPAA wellness program requirements is not determinative of compliance with the ADA. Therefore, in addition to HIPAA guidelines, you should consider the applicability of the ADA to your health management program during the design phase. You should seek legal guidance in designing and implementing such programs to ensure that they comply with ADA nondiscrimination requirements.

The ADA's wellness warning

It is important to note that the ADA provisions apply only to disabled individuals, which are defined by a physical or mental impairment that substantially limits one or more major life activities. Most behaviors targeted by wellness programs

do not rise to the level of a disability under the ADA, although obesity and stress-related disorders have sometimes been called into question as potential disabilities.

However, employers with health management programs must still be aware of those things that potentially violate ADA law, such as:

- Making participation in the wellness program mandatory

- Using information obtained in the program in a way that violates the ADA's confidentiality requirements

- Using information gained through the program to discriminate against employees who do not meet management's fitness expectations

In a question-and-answer session between The Joint Committee on Employee Benefits of the American Bar Association and representatives of the Equal Employment Opportunity Commission (EEOC), the EEOC provided informal insight into how the ADA applies to wellness programs. Its findings indicated that any wellness program requiring employees to answer disability-related inquiries, or submit to medical exams, must be on a voluntary participation basis. It also agreed that higher premiums or deductibles that penalize employees who don't cooperate were a violation of

ADA guidelines, because such premiums amount to penalties for nonparticipation and render participation in the program involuntary.

In terms of health risk assessments (HRAs), the conditioned enrollment in a health plan for participation in an HRA, which identifies certain risk factors, might render participation in the assessment involuntary. Many of these disability-related inquiries or medical exams, which are usually part of the assessment, are unlawful under the ADA.

As for exceptions, a voluntary wellness program exception statute reads, "A covered entity may conduct voluntary medical examinations, including *voluntary* medical histories, which are part of an employee health program available to employees at that work site."

The key to many ADA guidelines is emphasized in the word *voluntary*. Program participation must be voluntary to stay within legal constraints. Although the EEOC has not promulgated any regulation about the meaning of *voluntary*, the term means that no penalty can be imposed for not participating; and anything other than a de minimis incentive is prohibited.

From the preceding discussion of both HIPAA and the ADA, it is evident that there is sometimes conflicting information in the two laws. Other federal and state laws can complicate this further. There is a considerable amount of gray area, and companies are being left to interpret much of this for themselves. In our experience, how aggressive a company gets in structuring its health management program and offering incentives is often a factor of risk aversion and company culture, and its definition of *de minimis*.

Additional Legislation

Pending legislation for wellness programs is covered in a variety of bills that have been introduced in both the House and the Senate. Most of these are friendly to health management programs and, if enacted into law, would provide tax credits for companies that promote employee and dependent health, tax deductions for individuals for expenses related to maintaining good health, and additional research to support the value of health management. Some bills to watch that have been introduced as of June 2008 but have not yet been enacted into law include the following:

- Healthy Lifestyles Act (S. 2399)

- Healthy Workforce Act (S. 1753 and 1754)

- Help America Act (S. 2558)

- Workforce Health Improvement Program Act (H.R. 1818; S. 1491)

- Health Promotion First Act (S. 866)

With the growing popularity and proliferation of workplace health management programs, you can expect to see additional federal and state legislation in this area. Therefore, it is recommended that you stay abreast of any pending laws that may impact your health management initiatives going forward.

It is important to remember that compliance with HIPAA's nondiscrimination provisions does not reflect compliance with any other provision of ERISA, including COBRA's and ERISA's fiduciary provisions or other state or federal laws. It would be prudent to check with your human resources and legal departments in these areas to make sure your health management program continually meets HIPAA guidelines, as well as complying with other legal requirements.

State Laws

Certain state laws protect the confidentiality of employees' medical information and may have ramifications on how you can request and collect employee health data. These laws most likely place limitations on the disclosure of medical information generated by a health management program. Your local state and regional laws may impact how you operate your health management initiative, so make sure to check local health statutes and with the Department of Labor to ensure compliance.

Also be aware that 20 states and territories now have "Smokers' Rights" legislation on the books that protect some behaviors of people who smoke.

As an example, Indiana's law states: "An employer may not . . . require as a condition of employment, an employee or prospective employee to refrain from using; or . . . discriminate against an employee with respect to the employee's compensation and benefits or terms and conditions of employment based on the employee's use of tobacco products outside the course of the employee's or prospective employee's employment" (Ind. Stat. 22-5-4-1).

You will want to check to make sure your health management program does not violate these laws. The 20 states and territories are Arizona, Connecticut, the District of Columbia, Indiana, Kentucky, Louisiana, Maine, Missouri, Mississippi, New Hampshire, New Jersey, New Mexico, Oklahoma, Oregon, Rhode Island, South Carolina, South Dakota, Virginia, West Virginia, and Wyoming.

Eleven states also currently have Lawful Conduct/Lawful Products laws. As an example, New York law states, "It shall be unlawful for any employer or employment agency to refuse to hire, employ or license, or to discharge from employment or otherwise discriminate against an individual in compensation, promotion or terms, conditions or privileges of employment because of: . . . an individual's legal use of consumable products prior to the beginning or after the conclusion of the employee's work hours, and off the employer's premises and without the use of the employer's equipment or other property." The 11 states are California, Colorado, Illinois, Minnesota, Montana, Nevada, New York, North Carolina, North Dakota, Tennessee, and Wisconsin.

Although in general no laws prohibit health management programs, legislation such as HIPAA, the ADA, and various state and local laws have significant bearing on health plan eligibility and use of incentives. Many of the issues raised by these laws can be complex and multifaceted.

However, voluntary programs that allow all employees to participate and that provide incentives based solely on participation are rarely called into question by the laws. Still, it is wise to consult expert legal advice in matters requiring legal interpretation on any of these guidelines before beginning a companywide health management program. By doing so, you can avoid costly litigation, while providing your employees a healthy and supportive environment for maintaining their overall well-being.

Chapter 8

Evaluating Your
Health Management Program

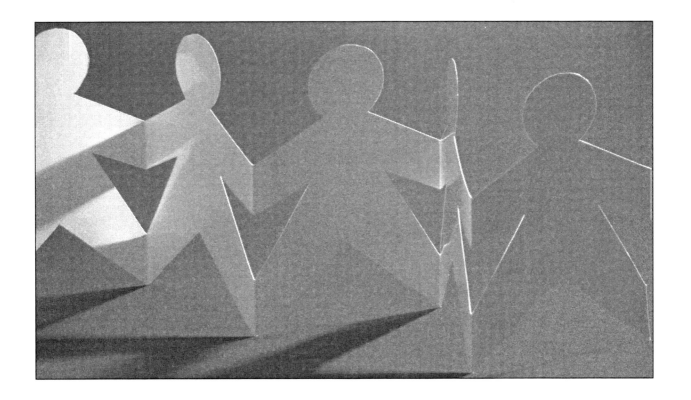

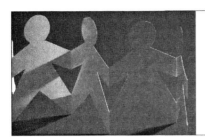

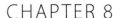

CHAPTER 8

Evaluating Your
Health Management Program

Program evaluation is critical in understanding the value and effectiveness of your health management program. To fully comprehend the impact your wellness program is having on your employees and dependents and health-related cost, you need to track and collect a variety of measurements and data. These include participation levels, employee satisfaction surveys, reductions in risk factors, changes in health behavior, and cost/benefit analyses. Ultimately, you should analyze and report the findings for each of these, and then aggregate the data.

The evaluation process will also allow you to glean information valuable in creating continuous quality improvement of your program and in maintaining executive support for the program. It is vitally important that you collect and report the right information to ensure the ongoing success of your company's initiatives.

Program evaluation serves a number of valuable functions. These include:

- Validating the decision to develop and launch a program in the first place

- Providing the evidence your company needs to continue supporting (or expanding) the program

- Providing ongoing measurement of the effectiveness of various program components

- Helping to make necessary modifications and adjustments to the program design

- Justifying the need and expenditure for outside vendor services

At its heart, a solid evaluation plan permits you to see whether the health management program is working the way you planned. It will give you the evidence you need to determine whether the program is meeting goals and objectives, and the ability to compare various program components for effectiveness. Other critical questions a good evaluation program can answer include the following:

- Is participation meeting objectives? If not, why not?

- Are some departments of the company more involved in the program than others? Why?

- Are employees taking the health risk assessment (HRA)?

- What are some of the trends that are being noted in the screenings and assessments?

- Did the in-person and telephone coaching have a measurable impact on behavior change?

- Are certain programs succeeding more than others? If so, why?

- Are the incentives working to achieve their objective, or do we need to modify the rewards offered?

- Has our culture support for health improved?

- Can we measure return on investment (ROI)?

By taking baseline measurements before the beginning of the program, you can effectively measure improvement over time, and show cause and effect. Your evaluation effort should access employee attendance, sick leave usage, employee turnover, and other productivity-related impact. You can also access overall healthcare usage.

Although evaluation is time-consuming and costly, it is an essential part of your health management program. It will bring forth some valuable insights immediately, while others will only be measured over time. When effectively conducted, your evaluation effort will yield ongoing support for the program, and become an essential business tool.

Evaluation Preparation

Evaluation involves using the data collected to determine if you have your goals and objectives. Keep in mind that simply collecting data does not constitute evaluation, although you cannot evaluate without the data.

To begin evaluation preparation, it is wise to put key components in place. To start, identify the staff members who will be involved in the evaluation process and its design. Make sure they understand how the evaluation process will be analyzed and administered. You must do this before the health management program is launched so the proper data is collected, stored, and reported.

A key decision that must be made is what database will be used to store the information. Some organizations create their own, while others contract for database services through data warehouse companies or major universities. Once a database is selected, it must be determined how claims, programmatic, and participant eligibility data will flow into the database. Finally, you must determine what will be evaluated and reported on a regular basis.

It is important to clearly determine what you want to evaluate and report on regularly. Modifications can be made over time as more is learned. Early in the program, you may want to focus on early indicators of success, while later in the program you may want to focus on more longitudinal outcomes.

Remember that:

- Participation drives behavior change

- Behavior change eliminates risk factors

- Reduced risk factors result in reduced incidence of illness and injury

- Reduced incidence of illness and injury results in reduced cost and higher worker productivity

Behavior change is what you seek, particularly as applied to the "Big 10": five modifiable lifestyle-related risk factors and five early detection/screening measures for adults:

Lifestyle:

- Tobacco

- Aspirin use for men over age 40 and women over age 50

- Alcohol use in moderation

- Nutrition and weight control

- Physical activity

Screening:

- Hypertension screening and treatment

- Cholesterol screening and treatment

- Breast cancer screening for women over age 40

- Colorectal cancer screening for adults over age 50

- Cervical cancer screening for women

It is widely recognized that the five lifestyle risk factors mentioned account for more than 80% of the chronic disease burden in the United States.

Measuring participation in programs that impact these 10 areas and ultimately the success you have in reducing these risk factors will tell you much about the early success of your health management effort.

You will need to track your costs in addition to outcomes. It is essential to have accurate program costs to calculate a meaningful ROI for your initiative.

You will often be asked to justify program expansion based on your outcomes and your ROI results. To resonate with management, your outcomes should be stated in concrete terms and they should address both health and cost/benefit information.

Finally, you will need to have a strategic communications plan in place to share the evaluation results with all key stakeholders. While presenting program results to management is essential in maintaining program support, employees at all levels should be informed about the program's overarching results. Inviting your workforce to see program results will encourage greater buy-in and will yield more participation in the initiatives. Results can be communicated through the same channels as you used to announce and promote the program.

Keep in mind that the overall objective of evaluation is to measure whether your disease management and wellness programs are effective in achieving your program goals. In addition, the evaluation plan can help to determine the resources and expertise needed to execute the program, and to balance outcomes against program cost to achieve an acceptable ROI.

Accomplishing Your Program Objectives

As we mentioned, to have an effective health management program, you must establish various objectives and measure them over time to determine whether the program is achieving its mission. You will need to understand whether the program is achieving desired results and, if not, what modifications need to occur to make achievement possible. Some of these objectives could include:

- Changing or improving employee health habits

- HRA participation penetration

- Reducing employee/dependent health-care costs

- Reducing workers' compensation and disability cost

- Reducing emergency room visits

- Reducing absenteeism and turnover

- Achieving smoking cessation

- Striving to maintain ideal weight among employees

- Increasing employees' level of physical activity

- Improving productivity and especially presenteeism

- Sustaining these improvements over time

Using multiple measures is required to assess the overall effectiveness of your program. In terms of collecting baseline data, one of the best measurement instruments is the HRA. Encouraging as many employees as possible, usually with some form of an incentive, to take the HRA will reveal some of the most useful baseline data for evaluation of employee health habits and personal lifestyle preferences over time.

HRAs should be reported at regular intervals, such as annually. Ideally, you should see improvement in people taking two consecutive HRAs at the first interval. A commonly used approach to assessing improvement across a population is to aggregate HRA and biometric results for people taking the consecutive HRAs to create an index score of total health risk. Biometric risk factors that can be tracked includes blood pressure, cholesterol (HDL and LDL), conitine (a byproduct of nicotine used to access exposure to tobacco), body mass index, glucose, as well as various self-reported lifestyle behaviors. The objective is to see the net risk in the population drop over time, with improvement in each risk category.

Another metric sometimes used to evaluate the effectiveness of a health management program is a review of employee productivity. It is advisable to measure absenteeism, which is one component of productivity, throughout the organization before and after program launch, if possible. However, this can be complicated. For instance, employers may be absent on any given day for myriad reasons other than illness, particularly in an era of personal time off (e.g., sick child, graduation of spouse or child, attending a funeral or wedding, and jury duty). Presenteeism, another component of productivity, is typically even more difficult to quantify. This is especially true for knowledge workers. The measurement of attention span and how well decisions are being made based on worker health status and similar factors is complicated.

Fortunately, tools such as the HPQ-Select, developed by Dr. Ron Kessler at Harvard University, are available for use separately or can be built into an HRA to capture productivity data without making these assessments too lengthy or complicated.

Adding workers' compensation and disability claims into the evaluation of your health management program may yield even more information on the value of your initiative. Reviewing your organization's workers' compensation or disability data may identify specific concerns within departments. For instance, if the evaluation of the data shows a spike in loading-dock employees filing workers' compensation claims for back pain, you can take specific action to address the issue through safety and wellness initiatives. Over time, if you address these specific issues through your health management program you should experience a reduction in workers' compensation and disability insurance claims.

In addition to what has been addressed here, you can target other factors specific to your workforce. Every organization must take the time to understand what it wants to measure, and how. Although there are commonalities that transcend organizations, you must still recognize that what makes sense for one organization may not work for another. Without this preliminary forethought, your data collection and outcomes evaluation might miss the intended mark.

Good participation rates and program effectiveness leads to risk factor reduction, a reduction in the incidence of illness and injury, and improvements in productivity. An effective health management program will have measurable impacts on greater employee satisfaction.

Conducting a Culture Audit

Before launching your health management program, we advised you to conduct a culture audit. A companywide health culture audit measures an organization's overall culture in terms of health and productivity, and can provide valuable feedback from your employees on their perception of the company's commitment to health and well-being.

With the initial data from the original culture audit, you can repeat the process once your health management program is well underway and compare responses. This approach is valuable because of the personal responses and anecdotes you will receive. This second audit can also assist you in making any policy changes that you might deem necessary for your company. Because you will have objective information from the evaluation, along with the additional support of the culture audit, you will have the justifications you may need for these policy changes, instituting premium differentials, or subsidizing the purchase of healthy food in your corporate cafeteria.

Evaluating Program Administration

When evaluating the program's progress, you must consider how effectively the program is being marketed and administered. Your evaluation process should determine effectiveness of program administration, and delivery. Although outcome data can certainly paint a picture of how a program is being operated, feedback will be equally valuable to weighing program effectiveness.

Some questions that you may want to answer in the survey include the following:

- Was there a high level of program awareness? Was communication effective and understandable?

- Did the program effectively reach those employees in greatest need?

- Did health habits improve?

- Did large numbers of employees participate in the program?

- Did the program achieve high employee satisfaction?

- Were incentives fairly granted? Were incentives desirable?

By evaluating your employees' awareness of and satisfaction with the program, you can better understand the actions necessary to improve the program over time. The responses to this survey will help you better determine whether the program is communicated effectively and is understood by end users. The survey can also solicit valuable feedback regarding the reasons for employee nonparticipation, which could prove to be most beneficial of all. If you want to get specific about the lack of participation, the survey can provide reasons for an employee to check off, such as the following:

- I was unaware of the program

- I am not motivated enough to participate

- I don't trust the confidentiality of the HRA

- The class locations are too far away from my work site

- Programs are not scheduled at convenient times for me

- I worry that my health information will be known by my employer

- I have trouble arranging for transportation to activities

- I am not interested in the class or lunch topics

- The exercise classes and equipment are inadequate to fit my needs

- I am self-conscious about addressing my health concerns with others

- I am not interested in the incentives offered

You should design these questions to measure what is most important for your organization. Through sustained participation, you will know whether your program is successfully addressing your workers' needs.

Tracking participant satisfaction with the program activities, classes, incentives, materials, exercise facilities, and anything else provided can be one of the most telling evaluation measurements. Therefore, administering an employee satisfaction survey and allowing employees to freely express their likes and dislikes can provide the kind of in-depth information that is needed to make the modifications to bring satisfaction rates to high levels. You can gather participant satisfaction responses throughout the year by providing evaluation forms to be completed right after various classes and lunch programs. Then consider conducting an employee satisfaction survey for the program as a whole every six to 12 months.

Developing an Evaluation Timeline

Because routine reports and updates are critical in monitoring the direction and needs of your health management program, you will need to develop a working timeline for evaluation and reporting that allows for dissemination to senior management and the employee population. Because some program objectives will be accomplished within a few months and others will take much longer, management will need a timeline to track and communicate what goals and objectives are being met.

Reporting can begin as soon as the program launches. Some information can be reported weekly or monthly, while others quarterly or annually.

A carefully planned timeline for reporting will permit you to consistently evaluate outcomes, which is critical in keeping your wellness program on track. It will also keep your evaluation efforts in process. Finally, it will set expectations for the organization on when all types of information will be evaluated and reported.

If performed properly, evaluation will help you demonstrate the costs and benefits associated with your health management program and where those costs and benefits occurred. Regular evaluation also allows you to make period-to-period comparisons much more easily, particularly in light of any benefit changes that may have been instituted.

All of the data collected and evaluated over time (year-to-date, year-over-year, and historical) has value, whether it results in positive or negative findings. The purpose of evaluation is to seek the

trust and to learn from it. As was discussed earlier, if the organization has made employee health part of its corporate mission, program results may even appear in the annual report. Other places in which results could be communicated include the company's internal and external newsletters, press releases, and even shareholder and community meetings.

Finally, once a critical mass of data is available, the executive steering committee should perform a formal review. Questions to be addressed include:

- Does the steering committee believe the program is meeting the needs of employees and senior management?

- Is the health and financial impact data compelling?

- What course corrections might be recommended?

- Is the steering committee doing all it can to support a culture of health?

If conducting your own evaluation is beyond your capability or you would prefer to outsource it, you can get assistance from outside parties that specialize in this. Most have created tools and processes, but the ability to transfer eligibility, participation, claims, and outcomes data electronically is still required. Consulting groups, database houses, and major universities often have this capacity.

Whichever way you decide, keep in mind how important the tracking of results and evaluation of outcomes is to the program's success. In time, you will find that evaluation is what drives continuous quality improvement, and optimizes the impact of your health management program.

Chapter 9

Revitalizaing a Stagnant
Health Management Program

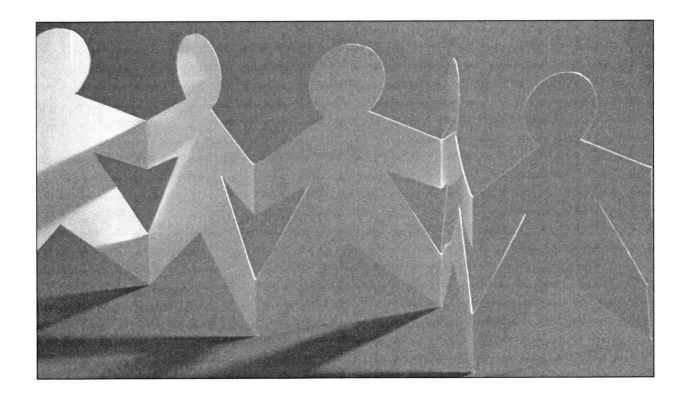

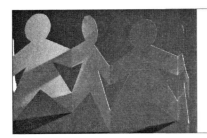

Revitalizing a Stagnant Health Management Program

In earlier chapters, we stressed the importance of carefully planning your health management program. A prudent approach to your organization's initial foray into health management is to establish a strategy that will provide some easy wins. Using such an approach can often help you avoid the headache of having to revitalize a program that is performing below expectations. However, if your organization has a health management program that is lagging in participation, there are ways you can revitalize employee interest and involvement. By following the processes, procedures, and philosophy that we have outlined in this book, you can rebuild your wellness program to the level you would like to achieve. We urge you to go carefully through this book and methodically put the components in place that will recharge your program. Here are some of the most important points.

Evaluate Your Current Health Management Program

To determine where your current effort stands within the organization, you need to perform a thorough evaluation of the existing program. Without such an evaluation, it will be difficult to pinpoint where changes and modifications need to take place.

There are three potential likely sources to review if the program is not meeting objectives. These include:

- Management support and assimilation of health into the corporate culture

- Program failure

- Inadequate program evaluation

To some extent whether or not there is management support for the health management program is obvious.

- Is the executive steering committee functioning?

- Has employee health become part of the corporate mission?

- Has a culture audit been conducted and actions taken?

If the answer to any of these questions is "no," lack of management or cultural support may be a big part of the problem.

As we have discussed, program evaluation is critical in understanding the value and effectiveness of your health management program. To fully comprehend the impact your current wellness program is having or not having, you should track a variety of measurements and collect the resultant data. This includes participation levels, employee satisfaction surveys, risk factor reductions, changes in health behavior and outcomes, and cost/benefit analyses.

Evaluating how employees feel about how the program is being marketed and administered is also crucial to the evaluation process. Your evaluation process should include specific measurements to determine and evaluate the program administration, as well as a survey of all workers to gauge their *perception* of the program.

By surveying your employees' awareness of the program, you can better understand the knowledge of existing programs, the kinds of activities employees want, and the best methods for enrolling workers and keeping them motivated over time. The responses to this survey will help you better determine whether the program is communicated enough and is understood by everyone. The survey can also solicit valuable feedback regarding the reasons for employee nonparticipation.

Tracking participant satisfaction with the program activities, classes, incentives, materials, exercise facilities, and anything else provided can be one of the most telling evaluation measurements. In fact, the perception employees have of the health management program can literally make or break its success and directly impact its continuation.

If your program is not where you want it to be in terms of participation or outcomes, understanding this perception is important. Therefore, administering an employee satisfaction survey and allowing employees to freely express their current likes and dislikes can provide the kind of in-depth information needed to make the modifications that will bring satisfaction, and participation rates and outcomes to higher levels.

Where to Start?

Assessing the level of senior management involvement is key and should be your starting point. Additionally, in parallel you should conduct an assessment of your steering committee members to gather their perceptions. This may have to take the form of a self-assessment, particularly if the steering committee has been tasked with conducting the overall evaluation.

The goal is to identify the root cause, if at all possible, for their lack of commitment and subsequent poor involvement. It is particularly important to tease out and to understand what led to their lost interest, if they were initially committed to the initiative. The bottom line is that you need to understand at a deep level what's behind the sentiment.

Once you have this information and understanding, you can help your steering committee move forward with the next steps. However, *do not* move forward until you are satisfied that you have identified the root causes that led to the failure the first time.

Many organizations struggle in being honest with themselves and dealing directly with the issues that caused them to fail. With that said, this is also the point of greatest potential growth for the organization. Indeed, it should be embraced as a major learning opportunity.

Many factors may point to why your health management program is stagnating. The following lists the likely next steps that an organization should consider if it is faced with the task of revitalizing an initiative on the verge of collapse:

1. Survey the executive team and steering committee:

   a) It is important to capture their definition for success

   b) Revisit the initiative charter (its mission/vision)

   c) Re-commit to making health part of the corporate vision

2. Survey and interview participants and nonparticipants:

   a) Questions should be designed to uncover specific issues. Generic feedback is not what is most useful in this situation.

   b) Nonparticipant perceptions can be invaluable in learning how to market your program in the future.

3. Restrategize and plan appropriately

4. Reexecute

Determine Executive Management and Employee Support

The support of executive management, especially the president or CEO, is vital in establishing a culture of health and building a strong program relaunch. In addition to executive management, supervisors and managers will also play an integral role in the success of the program. Employees look for leadership and support from management. If workers see executives and managers wholeheartedly embracing a culture of health, they too will be more inclined to participate. If your wellness program's participation has waned, check to see what message executive management is sending about its importance.

We have found that a lack of executive support often lies at the heart of this lack of participation. We have pointed out how critical the support of executive management can be in launching and maintaining a health management program. We have also emphasized throughout this book that without this support, the program may never get off the ground, or may languish from lack of participation.

One way to avoid this is to get commitments from various department heads, and other respected leaders in the organization, particularly if they have had a role in the past in representing or overseeing various components of the health management program. Without these commitments, enthusiasm for the program may wane, especially when seemingly more-pressing matters arise.

Plan Appropriately for Future Success

Appropriately planning for the future entails basing your strategic direction on sound information. Only then will you really know where to make the necessary program changes in design and delivery.

Getting back on track can mean taking the time to

rethink the goals and objectives of the program and then developing a realistic timeline for improvement.

As you plan, keep in mind some common reasons that programs falter:

- Lost sight of the original program vision and mission

- Poor communication and misguided expectations

- Lack of appropriate rewards and incentives

- Failure to establish a genuine culture of health within the organization

- Inadequate resources (budget and personnel)

- Poor planning

- Poor implementation

Conduct surveys and interviews

As we discussed in Chapter 2, your company should conduct initial surveys or companywide focus groups to determine the awareness and receptivity to your current wellness program. When programs stall, essentially you must start from the beginning to understand why. This requires that you look back at your initial survey findings and compare them with your new findings.

Certainly, at this point you also want to use all the program-specific performance data available, as well as existing health data. This information can reveal important facets needed to either relaunch or modify the existing program. This is a luxury you didn't have when you first launched and you should fully utilize it in your relaunch to avoid making the same or similarly costly mistakes.

One-on-one interviews with various department heads, senior executives, and other employees can also yield valuable feedback that can help to bring cohesion to the planning process. Some examples of questions to ask include the following:

- Are you currently participating in the health management program? Why or why not?

- What do you like best about the program?

- Did you take the health risk assessment (if one was provided)?

- What do you think of the incentives and rewards? Are they distributed fairly?

- Is the online technology associated with the program helpful?

- Do you feel the program is communicated effectively throughout the organization?

- Do you feel senior management is actively involved in the wellness program?

- Do you feel the organization gives its "permission" for employees to attend to their personal health?

- What suggestions would you make to improve the program?

By asking your employees whether they are participating in the program and how they feel about the program, you can gather important perceptions about the changes and modifications needed to make your program an enthusiastic success.

Once you have determined the program's initial direction, you can create a strategic plan of action, following the steps we have outlined in this book. This plan of action should start with the creation of a vision statement, mission statement, and goals and objectives for the program.

Revisit the initiative charter (mission and goals)

Many health management programs falter because the organization loses sight of its original vision and mission. Executives, managers, and employees are so busy with their jobs and other obligations that they fail to fully accomplish your goals. Frequent review of your objectives with senior leadership is vital. You should use every opportunity to seek clarity of mission and feedback of how others perceive the program is performing. The frequency factor helps to dispel misconceptions that, if held too long without being challenged or corrected, can fester. The program, of course, becomes the casualty.

A lack of a clear mission can impact the program's success. If one does not exist or if it's ambiguous or no longer accepted by leadership, now is the time to develop a new mission statement for the program. You can fold your program mission into company's values, ideals, and standards so that they reflect the principles that highlight the company's reasons for doing business. This approach can boost the credibility of the program while demonstrating a commitment to the long-term health and well-being of your workers.

It's no secret that employees at all levels will feel more attuned to a wellness program if it caters to their individual health needs, while meeting the corporate mission. The combination of specific goals and objectives, combined with the flexibility of allowing employees to achieve reasonable success, will enhance participation and, ultimately, the program's success.

Reexamine your program's rewards and incentives

As we've discussed, motivating workers to make lifestyle changes can be a challenging undertaking. It has demonstrated that companies that motivate employees to make positive behavior changes will experience better results than those that do not.

If you notice a drop in enrollment or participation in your health management program, scrutinize your incentives and reward program to see whether modifications can bring new enthusiasm. We outlined how to develop an effective incentives program in Chapter 2. Like your overall wellness program, your incentives and rewards component will need structure, goals, and objectives. You will need to determine what kinds of behaviors will be rewarded and how.

This is a good opportunity to seek employee feedback, especially from employees involved in the program. Here are two possible questions to ask:

- How do you feel about the incentives and rewards currently offered?

- Is a lack of meaningful incentives one of the reasons the program has seen a decline in participation?

If employees feel that the incentive goals and objectives are unobtainable or unfair, they may reject the whole program. This may be a good reason for the lack of enthusiasm your program is experiencing.

As we illustrated, the kinds of incentives and awards given out are vital. Employees will more enthusiastically pursue rewards that are intrinsically important to them. You might consider talking with companies that specialize in providing ready-made rewards and incentives. They will give you ideas about the kinds of incentives to offer and may help with some strategic ideas for reenergizing your program with employees.

It's also important to remember that incentives that are tied to the benefit plan can mobilize workers and their dependents to improve their health, while controlling costs. People want to save money. Incentives that help employees become good consumers of effective healthcare services are an excellent way to control costs for both companies and individuals.

So, be mindful of the value that a fair and rewarding incentive component can have on your health management program.

Reassess the Use of Online Tools and Technology

As we discussed in Chapter 4, there are many ways to approach your health management program, but it can improve its reach and ease of delivery. Tools do not make the program. Regardless of the programs and initiatives you include in your program, an arsenal of online technology coupled with real-life tools can create a potent formula for success.

With these technologies and strategies in place, you will be able to implement ongoing behavior change programs that will have a significant impact on your employees. The advantage of

online tools and remote communications devices are that you will have a greater chance to engage your employees where they are. The majority of employees live very busy lives. It is difficult, if not impossible, to reach them by traditional means (i.e., by home telephone and printed materials). Therefore, when implemented and used successfully, these technologies can connect with and persuade employees to make the simple, day-to-day choices that can have lasting repercussions in their health.

Examine Your Budget and Staff Resources

Many health management programs either wither or never take off because of a lack of funds and proper staffing. Providing a sufficient budget to cover expenses and staffing is crucial to success. A program that was either not been properly funded from the beginning or is slowly starved of vital fiscal and personnel resources will have a difficult time making an impact on the organization and will eventually stall from neglect.

Does your current health program suffer from this problem? If so, and if you are serious about revitalizing the program, you must allocate sufficient funds and people to ensure its vitality. We have found a combination of internal and external resources to be the most effective approach in launching or relaunching the program.

As we discussed in Chapter 2, the steering committee should determine the additional personnel, program material costs, IT financial support, and outside vendor costs that will be needed for a successful program relaunch. You will also need to determine whether existing staff members can handle the added responsibilities and demands of a revitalized health management program. That, in fact, may be a big part of the problem. Are people too busy to fulfill their roles?

If the organization makes a health culture the centerpiece of its health management program, you will have an easier time getting funds and getting people enthusiastically involved. This will also help in effectively supporting positive health habits. Without this change in perspective, your health program may never reach its potential.

We want to stress that funding your wellness program lies at the heart of its continued success. If the company is reluctant to put enough money into the program, consider what it will cost down the line if your employees do not embrace health. It will be far more affordable to help your workers maintain their health than it will be to get them healthy after they get sick.

Other departments in your organization have their own budgets, and would be far less expensive if inadequately funded. Think of your health management program in the same light. If your current health management program has stagnated, a

fresh infusion of money and people could be the first step in getting it back on track.

Hire Additional Staff Members, Consultants, and Outside Vendors

If you determine that additional staff members or outside consultants or vendors are needed to revitalize your health management program, hiring the needed people before the relaunch can help to ensure a success.

Most successful wellness programs have one person who oversees the day-to-day operations. Having this individual visible as the "face" of the program lends legitimacy, while also giving employees someone to go to if they have questions or require clarifications. If your current program lacks such a "face," consider appointing or hiring such a person.

You can also employ various outside vendors and consultants in helping you reposition and relaunch your in-house program. As we noted, these companies have experience in the realm of health management and can save you time and money. Utilizing them as a partner can help launch your program faster, easier, more effectively, and in many cases, with less cost than trying to do it all on your own. A preliminary check into what such a company can do for you should at least be a consideration, particularly if your program has languished.

Create a Realistic Timeline

Successfully relaunching your new health management program will be best achieved if it is not competing with other company events, product launches, national holidays, or other seasonal busy times. By removing the clutter of extraneous events and distractions, you will help your employees be focused on the relaunch.

Timelines, like goals, are most effective when documented. Creating an outline of critical dates and times may mean the difference between a focused and successful relaunch and a chaotic one. Employees who see a streamlined program, complete with set dates, will tend to want to participate in the program, especially when they see that the company has thought the new relaunch through.

To begin, break down each of your program's current components (assessments, coaching, data collection, etc.) and then calculate how long some of them will take to complete or redo. Although many parts of the program will be ongoing, some components will need to be completed within a finite amount of time at the beginning. Allow ample time to avoid being a victim of your own success. It is likely more people will participate this time, and thus you must anticipate and accommodate the increase.

Ask what specific tasks need resolution for each

part and when they need completion. Defining this kind of timeline will allow you to keep track of important start and stop dates while maintaining control over the entire process.

Revisit Your Communications Plan

A proper reintroduction and ongoing communication of your health management program will be vital to its success going forward. This is your new chance to reconnect and to raise awareness of the program—its importance and its value.

Your program should start with a new comprehensive marketing and promotion plan that is aimed at all of the organization's levels. The plan should recognize the organization's different constituencies. Buy-in from all of these groups will be necessary for a successful program. If you want "consumers" to engage in the relaunch you must effectively "sell" health management programming to workers and their dependents. Effective communication will maximize the chances that they will hear, understand, and, most importantly, act on the message.

One option you may want to consider is having an outside firm develop the program's communications plan. Both public relations firms and some health programming consulting groups can provide this service. The outsourcing of plan development can save staff time and help keep the relaunched wellness program on schedule.

Promoting the health management program message must become the rule, not the exception. One way to achieve this is the ongoing use of existing company communications to promote the health management program, such as in-house newsletters, benefits communications, safety communiqués, and broadcast e-mails or voice mails. Without these, the new program will suffer. A well-planned effort continually utilizing these resources can be effective and cost-efficient.

Additionally, having an endorsement from the company president or other senior executive will lend credibility to the new program. A quarterly update by senior managers on progress, new programs, and other pertinent information can keep the program top of mind for employees.

Relaunch the Program

Once you have most of the program's components in place, it will be time to relaunch. The best way to achieve this is through a phased-in approach, especially if parts of the program are being offered to a subset of the work force.

If you begin with the program areas that are easiest and most likely to succeed, you can give employees an early win. Encourage flexible scheduling so that employees can participate fully. Online tools, sign-up sheets, record logs, and any other program materials should be readily available and located where employees will have easy access to them.

Issuing a letter from the CEO or president announcing the program's launch to every employee will underscore the importance of health throughout the organization. Recognizing the value that senior management places on the program may also induce more employee participation.

Make sure everyone in the organization understands who the program's leaders are and how the program works. This effort should also be part of the overall communications plan.

As the program is rolled out, encourage feedback from all levels of the company. Workers involved with the relaunch will have valuable insight into creating a more appealing program. As the program progresses, try to make incremental changes according to the feedback, until the program becomes completely integrated in the company culture. Although this may take time, these small changes can yield huge rewards. If you undertake these steps now, you will avoid having the program languish again.

Make Ongoing Evaluation a Priority

We thoroughly discussed how to evaluate an ongoing health management program in Chapter 8. Those steps and recommendations apply to the relaunch of a wellness program, too. As your new program unfolds, watch for ongoing developments, new ideas, creative approaches, and legal changes.

Remember that a health management program is designed as an external motivator until the true value of healthy behaviors is internalized. Ultimately, the key to success in creating and maintaining a health management program is to keep it simple, communicate it effectively, set up efficient program administration, and ensure the confidentiality of all participants.

Modify or Change the Program

Once you evaluate the data collected and answer some of these questions, you may decide that your new health management program still needs adjustment. This is to be expected. These programs are ever-changing. Adopting a flexible, phased-in approach to these changes will make them less disruptive and more effective.

Each chapter of this book should help in the modification process. We have detailed areas that you need to consider and implement to create an effective program. Taken as a whole, each chapter should help you make the small or large changes needed to develop the kind of health management program that will meet the needs of all employees.

Chapter 10

The Future of Workplace
Health in America

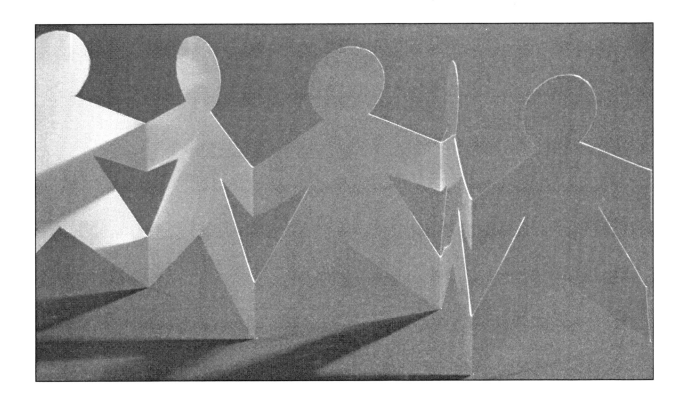

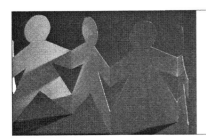

The Future of Workplace Health in America

Over the past 10 years, the fields of disease management and wellness in the United States have exploded. Of particular note is the trend of delivering disease management and wellness as part of an integrated health management strategy. When properly designed and delivered, health management efforts can become an important part of a business management strategy and can be fully embedded in the corporate business culture.

The growth of integrated health management programs has been driven by the escalating healthcare costs that are largely a result of an increase in lifestyle-related chronic illnesses. More recently, corporate America has also become increasingly concerned about the impact of poor health on worker productivity. Despite the fact that millions of people have embraced healthy habits, millions more have failed to act responsibly.

With the cost of healthcare impacting profitability, and with poor productivity making many organizations less competitive in a global economy, companies across the United States have recognized a need to keep their employees healthy. Smart

companies recognize that because they assume the health-related risk, they will also have to take a leading role in avoiding or mitigating the cost, rather than relying on outside influences to effect changes in current health trends. In fact, we predict that companies will embrace health management initiatives as a vital and tactical strategy, and will work to create an environment that supports and rewards healthy behaviors as part of the corporate culture. Because of its potential and given the magnitude of the problem, the health management initiative should be viewed as a highly viable corporate business strategy.

These changes are driving a new recognition of the importance and potential value of health management efforts in the years to come. In the foreseeable future, we see many likely changes as the state of the art in behavior change and clinical management of chronic illnesses matures. This could result in many new and exciting solutions to the complicated problem of maintaining health, and it could produce considerably better results in controlling cost and optimizing productivity for the corporate sector.

A New Way of Thinking

Although much has been learned about how to create and sustain health behavior change and about how to most effectively optimize the health of people with existing chronic illnesses, the future approach to health management will require complete restructuring to be most successful. This restructuring will likely occur simultaneously with and as a part of efforts to revamp the U.S. healthcare system. Companies that do not embrace new health management models for their workers may find themselves being less competitive in both the U.S. and global marketplaces, which will demand cost-efficient operations and highly productive workers.

The senior leaderships of both large and small companies alike are expressing concerns about how poor employee health will affect their organizations. Many have made major commitments to their health management strategies while others have at least begun to define their strategies and set priorities. As an example, in a survey conducted in 2007 by Hewitt Associates and titled *The Road Ahead: Emerging Health Trends*, employers indicated the following as their top three business issues:

- Managing costs

- Competitive positioning

- Profitability

They indicated these as their top three work force issues:

- Employee satisfaction

- Protecting employees against catastrophic health losses

- Improving productivity

From this information, it is evident that employers are looking for wellness-oriented solutions that are coordinated with disease and care management solutions.

Over the past 20 years, we have seen a shift from treating disease to preventing disease. However, much of that shift was directed toward tertiary prevention, preventive actions that occur after a person already has an illness. Thus, although it was a movement toward prevention, much of the strategy was still focused on people with illnesses. Even wellness programs have largely focused on secondary prevention, with efforts aimed at people with risk factors. Only recently has there been a significant focus on primary prevention, whereby the objective is to keep healthy and risk-free people in their current state.

In reality, as we discussed in Chapter 4, all types of prevention are important if we are going to have a major impact on the health of the entire population. This powerful paradigm shift will create both challenges and opportunities and will require a need for strategic thinking, thorough planning, careful design, and effective interventions and implementation. The shift will also require senior leadership to consider and act on what good health means to the company and its employees, and on how to best position the health of the organization for future strategic advantage.

The Trends Likely to Shape Our Future

A number of trends will likely shape the future of health management. In the following sections, we will address 12 of them.

Demographic shift

It is a well-known fact that America is aging. According to Experience Corps., the number of Americans age 55 and older will almost double between now and 2030, from 60 million today to 107.6 million. Furthermore, the number of Americans over age 65 will increase from 34.8 million in 2000 to 70.3 million in 2030. This shift in demographics not only will increase the prevalence of chronic disease, but will also change the way in which we deliver health management programs.

America is also becoming more disparate in race and ethnicity, and we are recognizing different needs of people of different races, ethnicities, and genders. Information and delivery systems that meet the needs of all demographic groups will be required. Further, a better understanding of the psychographic differences, preferred media, and other special needs and preferences of a demographically disparate population will be necessary. Efforts will also be required to address and remediate health disparities.

Culture

A sea change is coming in the way society sees and accepts poor health behaviors. A good example is how much the acceptance of smoking has changed over the past 30 years. Smoking is no longer accepted in most public places and is rarely allowed in the work environment. In fact, some companies have even taken steps to not employ smokers (where legal). If a smoker lights up in a restricted area, the consequences are predictable. Even people who are usually not confrontational immediately voice their displeasure.

Whether you believe it is right or not, some similarities are occurring with obesity. Americans appear to be losing tolerance for people who are overweight and are making no attempt to change. Even the Wellness provision in the Health Insurance Portability and Accountability Act of 1996 allows for legal discrimination against people who are overweight when it comes to incentive programming. Further, there are countless reports of hiring discrimination against the obese (though not legal). Although it may be unfortunate, overweight people are also the brunt of jokes and sometimes are seen as having inadequate discipline to change their situations.

On a more positive note, companies are realizing that they cannot possibly have a lasting impact on the health habits of their employees unless they create a supportive culture. Thus, many are embracing internal norms designed to be helpful. Stating the maintenance of good health and observing appropriate lifestyle habits as part of the corporate values or goals is a good place to start. Also, policies that prohibit smoking on work premises or that provide flexibility in work hours for exercising during the day helps to create the right environment. Providing healthy options in the cafeteria and access to exercise facilities also sets the right tone. Tools exist for measuring the extent to which the corporate culture is supportive of maintaining good health so that the organization can continually monitor its progress. All of these efforts increase the chances that employees and their dependents will choose to live a healthier lifestyle.

With societal pressure to observe good health and corporate initiatives to provide a supportive environment, it is likely that the public will experience a cultural shift away from unhealthy behavior (e.g., the three-martini lunch) and toward good behaviors such as exercise and good nutrition. This trend will help to impact health and its associated costs.

Changing delivery environments

How we serve up just about anything is changing. We read our newspapers online, we text-message our kids when it is time for them to come home, we instant-message instead of call people, and we telecommute. It is no longer unusual to conduct business in two different cities in the same day by simply flying from one place to another. We send e-mails instead of letters and expect almost instant return. To be successful, health management programs must keep pace.

Wellness programming has been mostly a large, self-insured company phenomenon, and there has been no coherent plan to deliver health management to the masses. Like electricity at the time of Thomas Edison, health management is a good concept. The question is, "How do we get it to 270 million Americans, let alone the rest of the world?" It is likely that delivery through aggregators will be at least part of the answer. Possible delivery sources include the following:

- **Health plans:** Health plans have shown promise because they reach the employees and dependents of even small companies. However, until recently they had not attempted to deliver health management services in any significant way. Although this is changing, chances are the health plans that are most successful will partner with health management vendors to produce the best results.

- **Third-party administrators:** Like health plans, third-party administrators have access to the lives of even small companies.

They have shown far less interest in serving up health management than health plans, and like health plans they will have the limitation of health management not being their primary line of business.

- **Chambers of Commerce:** Groups such as the local Chamber of Commerce can aggregate lives, but they still need to receive health management services from another party. However, they can help to reduce the cost of delivery through economy of scale.

- **Direct to consumer:** Direct to consumer actually shows significant promise. With consumer-driven health benefits has come the realization that employees and dependents may someday need to purchase prevention services on their own. Further, purchasing directly means that there are no issues with portability if an employee changes jobs or health plans. A number of entrepreneurial organizations have stepped forward to be of service. We will address these groups later in this chapter.

Although they have some limitations, employers are still the most likely sources of health management delivery. After all, they have the most to lose and gain. However, most companies also face delivery challenges. As workplaces become more fragmented, with employees telecommuting, working in virtual environments, and working split shifts, the health management programs of

the future will have to take these situations into consideration. In the future, companies will have to recognize and embrace the changing nature of work, and the work environment, and accommodate these in their health management programs. In other words, health management programs will have to be designed and tailored to fit the circumstances of employees. This will require more use of technology and flexibility in programming to reach the end-users where they live.

One final challenge employers will have to overcome is the globalization of their work forces. Advancement of health management beyond the United States will be necessary to treat all employees equitably, and to protect employees outside the United States. With most healthcare systems being different outside the United States, the program must emphasize productivity improvement more than medical care savings. Challenges will include reaching people some distance from the United States, programming in different languages, effectively addressing ethnic and cultural norms, and working with different healthcare systems and societal constructs.

Improved science

Although wellness programs have formally been in existence for more than 30 years, we still struggle to get people to make and sustain behavior change. Furthermore, we still struggle to understand the psychology of behavior change, or when it is equally effective to use pharmacotherapy or other forms of medical treatment to overcome physical problems when behavior change does not occur or is not enough. It is likely that over the coming years we will gain a greater understanding of how to most effectively treat behavior-related chronic illnesses using a combination of behavior change, traditional medicine, and complementary and alternative therapies.

Better understanding the psychology of behavior change shows promise. Research that has resulted in behavior change approaches, such as the Transtheoretical Change Model developed by Dr. James Prochaska, and the Compression of Morbidity Theory developed by Dr. James Fries, are examples. Furthermore, researchers such as Dr. Dee Edington have demonstrated the link between behavioral risks and cost. It is likely that advancement of the science and art of behavior change will improve our behavior change success rates, thereby reducing the incidence of illness and injury and, ultimately, disease-related cost.

Research in population management is likely to make us more effective in improving the health of large populations en masse. It may be improved science that helps us shift the thinking and actions of entire cultures toward embracing activities to promote well-being. One approach that shows great promise is social networking. As with Facebook, MySpace, and YouTube, health management pro-grams such as SilverSneakers and QuitNet have used social networking to help individuals support each other in their behavior change endeavors. It is likely that social networking will become a major part of the health support landscape.

Medical advances will continue that will help us better treat behavior-related chronic illnesses when they do occur. Also, a better understanding of genetics and when certain people are predisposed to chronic illnesses may help some become more committed to behavior change. Even bioengineering may play a role.

As in the past, the advancement of science will not come without some ethical questions. Should smoking be treated as an addiction or a failure to act responsibly? Is obesity a disability or a controllable condition? Should we use gastric bypass to treat obesity or focus primarily on behavior change? Should we use genetic testing in determining who receives certain types of medical care? Science has improved the quality of our lives in so many ways, but it also raises new ethical questions.

Legislative support for change

Legislation may play a role in the future of health management. A number of bills, if passed, could help to speed the transformation of health management. Here is a list of some of the laws that are pending:

- The Health Promotion First Act calls for better research in health promotion. This could fuel the interest of the political community and result in the funding of research that improves the quality of programming and a better understanding of health management program efficacy.

- The Healthy Workplace Act, if passed, would provide tax credits for employers offering qualified health management programs to employees. This could inspire even small companies to launch comprehensive health management initiatives.

- Several other bills are also pending, including ones that address personal tax credits for consumers purchasing fitness center memberships and ones that fund other health-friendly initiatives.

Legislation brings better visibility, credibility, and legitimacy to the health management field while also providing resources for change.

Better resources

A comprehensive health management program is expensive. It is impossible to solve a complex economic problem with a simple and inexpensive answer. To have any chance of success, the organization must provide significant fiscal support for the health management initiative. For the health management programs of the future to succeed, money will need to be earmarked for effectively

communicating, delivering, measuring, and evaluating the program. Anything less would be futile.

In recent years, many examples of companies that have dedicated significant resources to their health management efforts have emerged. These organizations are motivated by the belief that a well-developed and well-funded health management program will generate a return that exceeds the cost of the initiative. In the coming years, more companies will come to recognize the importance of properly funding the effort, because of the results that will be seen by the pioneers. This will result in greater programmatic success.

Health insurance reform

As we have seen in recent years, the cost of providing health benefits to U.S. employees is significantly eroding company profits, even for large corporations. Senior management, shareholders, and even the employees themselves are questioning the future viability of this path. In fact, many see this ongoing trend of rising healthcare expenses as going beyond reducing profits to actually threatening the long-range sustainability of companies that operate business as usual. As a result, the corporate and health plan sectors have become active with government to search for answers.

With a crisis at hand, many changes in healthcare law have been health-management-friendly. For instance, since 2002, when Congress made health savings accounts (HSAs) universally available, more than 3 million Americans have opened such accounts. Employers are now covering more than 6 million Americans with employer-sponsored health reimbursement arrangements, which allow employees to take a 100% income tax deduction for most wellness expenditures.

Other reforms are also likely, with more responsibility being shifted to the individual consumer and more active involvement of the government (state and federal). Although it is likely that employers will still bear the majority of the burden, the landscape will change, potentially impacting where the risk and opportunity for health management will fall. Therefore, companies must stay informed and be prepared to react to take advantage of new opportunities and to avoid unnecessary costs.

Finally, in the future, it is likely that health management initiatives will be routinely designed into the company's benefit plans. This will create the opportunity for a more integrated initiative and will also establish the appropriate linkage between benefits, disease management, and prevention. Preventive benefits and benefit-related incentives whereby employees pay less when they participate in appropriate prevention programs and activities will be part of this plan. It is even possible that compensation plans will be integrated in a way that encourages good health behaviors on the part

of employees, and rewards them for good behavior and results through additional compensation.

Value and accountability

An important and welcomed trend in health management is holding programs to a considerably higher level of accountability. Savvy employers, consultants, and health plans are better evaluating health management initiatives for participation, behavior modification, risk factor reduction, impact on medical care, and improvements in productivity and cost-effectiveness. Unlike in years past, today organizations must justify the value of health management programs to their management, boards, and shareholders, and thus, the vendors that deliver program components will not escape scrutiny.

To demonstrate value, good reporting is required. Reporting provides transparency so that the reader can best understand program outcomes.

A big part of ensuring value is performance guarantees. Clients are requiring providers of health management programs to guarantee certain outcomes of the program or face penalties. Performance guarantees are a reasonable expectation for vendors because of the substantial service fees corporate customers pay. However, a word of caution: Some purchasers of services are asking for guarantees on stretch goals, rather than on minimally acceptable performance. The industry reacts to unreasonable performance guarantee expectations by charging higher fees, falsely inflating prices. This can result in disappointment for all involved. Vendors are criticized for not meeting it, even though they knew that meeting the guarantee would not be likely, so they protected themselves with higher fees. The purchaser gets money back, but is criticized by its management, who would prefer performance rather than a rebate. So, performance guarantees are an important part of ensuring value, but their use needs to be sensibly applied.

It is likely that the way health management programs are charged will change significantly over the next five years. This will result in a change in how performance guarantees are used as well. Because people will move more fluidly through health management programs in the future, it will be more difficult to charge in the compartmentalized way health management vendors do now. At present, there is a per-participant fee, per-member per-month fee, or per-diseased-member per-month fee, depending on the program and the vendor. This works reasonably well because people tend to stay in the programs in which they are placed.

However, imagine a time when people move through the health management system based on their acuity each day, their learning style, their preferred media, and other factors. In such a model, people of all levels of health flow through a fully integrated model and are engaged at a nearly infinite number of touch points (we discuss this in

more detail later in this chapter). When that day arrives, charging for programming will become more complicated, as will administering some types of performance guarantees.

Because of the complications created by more sophisticated programming, in the future it is likely that pricing for health management programs will be based on pay per unit of value achieved, rather than fee for service. What that unit or units might be is yet to be determined. Likewise, it is possible that the percentage of achievement of unit of value will establish the amount a health management vendor gets paid. So, the methods of charging and performance guarantees will be combined into one. Such methods may even provide an upside for health management vendors if they exceed unit-of-value expectations.

These changes will require more sophisticated measurement of health management program outcomes. Expect significant changes in how success is measured as the science and the art become more sophisticated. Some of the data warehousing companies continue to make advancements in measurement, as do prominent universities. Industry support groups are also contributing. For instance, the Health Enhancement Research Organization Scorecard is a public domain program scoring system that has proven valuable in the industry. The National Committee for Quality Assurance has also developed standards for health management programs and most likely will develop others soon. Work has begun between Gallup and Healthways to establish a "Well-being Index" that could serve as the Dow Jones Industrial Average of health in the future. Expect rapid improvement in the sophistication of measurement of health management program value in the years ahead.

The focus on value will be good for corporations and their employees. It will also be good for health management service vendors. The most important thing at the end of the day is that the incentives for all stakeholders are aligned.

Highly integrated program delivery models

The effective delivery models of the future will be highly integrated. Unfortunately, the concept of integration has been discussed for several years, but little advancement has really occurred. Ask 10 people for their concept of integration and you will probably get 10 vastly different answers.

The models of the future will integrate data, programs, technologies, policies, cultures, and the actions of different types of professionals. Even information provided by participants through

their regular interaction with the health management system will be integrated with other data to provide the participant the ultimate personal experience. Individual participants, employers, healthcare providers, health plans, and specialized program vendors will all have a role. Figure 10.1 provides an idea of how an integrated framework might look.

In the model presented in Figure 10.1, a healthy environment is established for all individuals eligible for the health management program. Programs are provided to promote and support healthy lifestyles, to eliminate or reduce behavioral and biometric risk factors, and to optimize the care for people with chronic conditions. The employer is called upon to make health a corporate initiative, to develop and maintain a "Culture of Health," to establish business metrics that are linked to improved health outcomes, and to establish a health strategy that is incorporated into the corporate business objectives. A major action that many employers will take is to have health-friendly corporate policies and to design benefit plans that support good health behaviors, rather than just systematically paying for illness treatment.

Figure 10.1
Nontaxable and taxable benefits

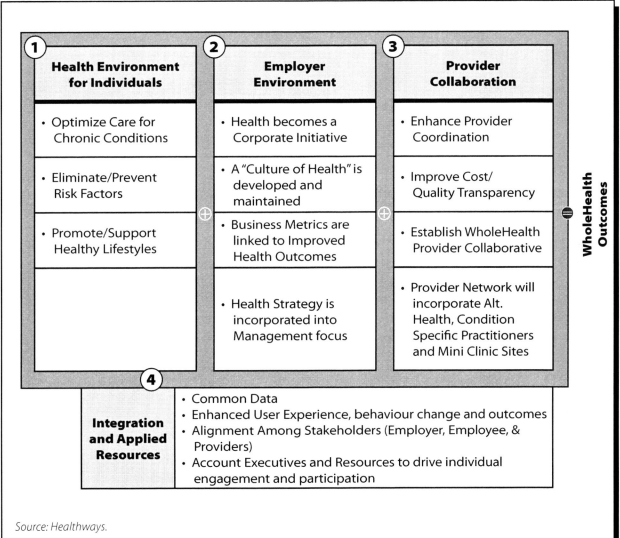

Source: Healthways.

In addition to the roles of individuals and employers, healthcare providers will also be called upon to do more. Provider collaboration like none that has ever existed will be necessary. A robust data system and targeted initiatives will enhance provider participation and coordination. Provider collaboratives, networks of alternative health practitioners, and on-site venues, such as fitness centers and mini clinic sites, will be integrated to maximize wellness impact.

All of this will be integrated through common data pooling, enhancing the user experience and better driving behavior change and outcomes.

The alignment of all stakeholders (employer, employees, health plans, providers, and service vendors) and the use of account executives and resources that drive individual engagement and participation will help to facilitate the success. When fully integrated, such a model will have a far-reaching impact on the population served, and may help the provider community as the public demands improved quality transparency, and pay-for-performance reimbursement systems gain popularity.

When the participant, healthcare providers, and support vendors all share the same integrated system and have visibility into the participant's information, health management efforts can be best coordinated. This provides continuous support to all participants. Instead of being treated like a smoker, a diabetic, or a person with obesity, the participant is treated as an individual with a unique set of needs that must be addressed.

Conceptually, it is likely that the way in which health management services will be delivered will also change. As stated earlier, people will move fluidly through the system on a just-in-time basis, receiving services on their terms. A combination of technology and human intervention will likely drive this change. In such a model, a professional will be responsible for a large group of people (say 5,000). Each day, technology will help the professional determine what services need to be provided to each person. For instance, people who

have been logging their exercise and weight regularly, and who appear to have everything under control, might receive a programmed congratulatory e-mail or text message that is system-generated.

On the other hand, people whose claims, interaction with a pharmacy, or recent doctor's visits indicate they have emergent needs might receive a phone call from a professional to receive immediate assistance. For people somewhere in between these two extremes, tailored outreach could occur. As an example, a person who has no known medical need but who has uncharacteristically ceased the use of the health management tools available might receive an e-mail reminder, a call, or even some form of a visit in an attempt to regain momentum. The system will apply the least expensive option of interaction, moving sequentially to higher-cost interventions if low-cost ones fail, all the time taking into consideration the participant's venue of preference as determined through previous interactions.

To be most successful, multiple coordinated/integrated venues to reach people must be used. These would include face-to-face visits, phone, Web, and mail. Also, virtual communities of support have shown promise and will likely be used more extensively in the future. Through these communities, participants with like needs and interests can help each other make and sustain behavior changes. It is also likely that communication will occur through a variety of vehicles that are gaining popularity, including PDAs, cell phone text messaging, Bluetooth uploads of information from devices such as pedometers, scales, and glucometers, and a variety of other devices with smart technologies.

The field of health management is currently fragmented in many ways. There are programmatic silos, and there is a lack of data consolidation and compatibility, no means for multiple service providers to communicate, total separation from the provider community, and an inability to coordinate between media venues. Integration has the potential to bring this together in the future, resulting in a coherent means of changing behaviors and supporting people on their health journey.

Targeted interventions

The integrated model just described has a direct impact on the individual participant. In fact, the system is designed to provide each participant with a unique experience specifically tailored to meet his or her needs. The system is designed to assess the participant using all known data and to design a personalized experience that:

- Supports healthy lifestyles

- Motivates participation to deliver the best health value

- Eliminates or improves risky behaviors

- Optimizes care for chronic conditions

- Delivers a personalize solution for improved health using the media and venues preferred by the participant

- Provides ongoing support

- Dynamically adapts as the participant does

The types of programs provided will include marketing and incentives to maximize participation, robust Web services that support participants in all of their health endeavors, networks of fitness centers and alternative health providers, health coaching, and disease management. More important, it will serve up and deliver these services in combinations that are totally unique for each participant.

Incentives

We have discussed the use of incentives in a number of other chapters, so we will provide less detail here. Suffice it to say that incentives will continue to be a part of the health management landscape in the future. It is likely that incentives will be used to drive participation in health assessments and interventions that maintain or improve health, as they have done in the past.

However, we expect more emphasis on providing incentives for improvement of objective biometric measures, such as cholesterol, blood pressure, and blood sugar, than we have seen in the past. We also expect continued focus on providing incentives for not using tobacco products, and in some cases using biometric measures, such as blood cotinine levels, to confirm nontobacco use status.

Although cash, benefit premium and copay deductions, enhanced contributions to HSAs, gift cards, and merchandise have all been used as incentives, it is likely that in the future most incentives will be directly tied to the benefit plan. Thus, it is expected that use of benefit cost reduction-type incentives will become more the norm.

Some of these incentives will become creative in nature, taking advantage of technology to track use of prevention services and other positive behaviors associated with the benefit plan. Leveraging incentives as part of the benefit plan sends a message to employees and dependents that there is a relationship between their behavior and the cost of the plan, and provides inducement to take responsibility for personal health habits and appropriate use of the healthcare system.

Although most incentives used today take a positive approach and thus apply the "carrot," it is likely that more incentive programs in the future will apply the "stick." There is a growing intolerance for having to reward people for doing the right thing. It is likely that this will instead lead to penalizing people for doing the wrong thing. Although the perception of such an approach may be less appealing, the use of the stick will probably be more cost-efficient and potentially more effective. Expect increased costs to be assessed to more than just smokers. Other behaviors, measureable biometric risks, and failure to participate in health improvement programs may also draw financial penalties.

Change fueled by consumer demand

Although much of America remains complacent about living healthy lifestyles, there is a growing demand for better services by people who have heard and are complying with the prevention message. These early adopters are looking for ways to make their quest to live a healthy lifestyle easier, more convenient, and more effective. This will result in several notable changes in how health management is delivered today.

As companies and individuals embrace the trend in wellness and disease prevention, the already growing wellness industry will expand even more. Wellness entrepreneurs have already begun to tailor specific products and services to an industry that is estimated at more than $500 billion.

Since its inception, the wellness industry has been considered a grassroots movement. However, all of that is changing. The wellness and disease management industry of today is clearly going mainstream, with the most significant growth and advancement probably still ahead. Experts predict that the industry will continue to grow for at least another decade, until wellness and disease management has become a mature industry, with a nearly saturated marketplace.

With wellness and disease management programs gaining legitimacy, new products, services, and even medical procedures will be developed. In fact, thousands of new health management products and services have already come to market, with thousands more likely to be under development but not yet identified. Many of these will leverage technology, whereas others will use improved science or delivery methods to maximize impact. Many new players will emerge while existing organizations will thrive.

However, over time many of these organizations will come together through mergers and acquisitions as consolidation occurs, as it does in any mature industry. In the meantime, both established entrepreneurs and new market entrants will drive the marketplace in bigger and more impactful ways than ever before, as they design more useful and successful health products and services.

It is also expected that a number of groups will enter the health management industry in ways not even imagined just a few years ago. For instance, retailers, especially health food stores and restaurants, will use the public's interest in wellness to gain market share. In the past, to find healthy foods one had to go to an "alternative"

health food store or an "alternative" restaurant. However, today many mainstream restaurants and food outlets, fast food franchises, and grocery stores are realizing the growing demand for healthy foods and are finding that providing healthy options can be good for their bottom lines.

As examples of how mainstream outlets are entering the wellness space, Wendy's and McDonald's now sell salads and fruit. In fact, in 2005, McDonald's became the largest food-service consumer of apples, requiring almost 54 million pounds per year. In 2006, Wal-Mart opened its first organic foods supercenter in Plano, TX, and began to sell wellness products in all of its stores. Dean Foods purchased WhiteWave, the maker of Silk soy milk, which it has continued to market as a wellness product. Safeway has a program called Foodflex that rewards loyal customers for making healthy purchases, and PepsiCo is promoting its Smart Choices program. Even Kellogg's, whose roots go back to providing nutritious food options, has added the Kashi brand to the other foods it manufactures.

These are just a few examples of the companies that have found value in embracing the wellness movement in America and abroad. It is likely that many more mainstream companies will embrace this consumer trend in the years ahead.

One final change that will continue as a result of consumer demand is the emergence of mini clinics in retail outlets. The latest entry into the retail clinic business is Walgreen's, which has entered through acquisition. As consumers seek a "health home," which is the center of what drives both their preventive and curative care, it is likely that they will look to what is convenient for them. Retail outlets are on the beaten path that consumers frequent each week, making them a good site for mini clinics. Thus, we anticipate that more care will be brought directly to the consumer, in his or her neighborhood, or even directly to his or her residence.

A Future Business Strategy

With health-related expenditures being one of the highest operating costs of most organizations, the implementation of an effective health management program can prove to be a highly effective business strategy. More and more organizations throughout the United States are implementing robust health management programs, and we expect the trend to continue. Many of the trends discussed in this chapter should be considered in providing a highly effective health management effort.

In the final analysis, organizations of the future are going to find that integrating health and disease management initiatives into the company culture will be a business requisite. When done appropriately, such efforts will play a central role in the process of managing cost and leading the organization to a successful future.